MEDICAL
INTELLIGENCE
UNIT

MOLECULAR AND CELLULAR BIOLOGY OF MELANOMA

MEDICAL
INTELLIGENCE
UNIT

MOLECULAR AND CELLULAR BIOLOGY OF MELANOMA

Meenhard Herlyn, D.V.M.

The Wistar Institute
Philadelphia

R.G. LANDES COMPANY
AUSTIN

MEDICAL INTELLIGENCE UNIT

MOLECULAR AND CELLULAR BIOLOGY OF MELANOMA

R.G. LANDES COMPANY
Austin / Georgetown
CRC Press is the exclusive worldwide distributor of publications of the Medical Intelligence Unit.
CRC Press, 2000 Corporate Blvd., NW, Boca Raton, FL 33431. Phone: 407/994-0555.
Submitted: March 1993
Published: May 1993
Production Manager: Judith Kemper
Copy Editor: Constance Kerkaporta

Please address all inquiries to the Publisher:
R.G. Landes Company, 909 Pine Street, Georgetown, TX 78626
or
P.O. Box 4858, Austin, TX 78765
Phone: 512/ 863 7762 FAX: 512/863 0081

ISBN 1-879702-55-X
CATALOG # LN0255

Library of Congress Cataloging-in-Publication Data
Herlyn, Meenhard.
Molecular and cellular biology of melanoma/Meenhard Herlyn.
p. cm.—(Medical intelligence unit)
Includes bibliographical references and index.
ISBN 1-879702-55-X (hard) : $89.95
1. Melanoma--Molecular aspects. 2. Melanoma--Cytopathology.
3. Melanoma--Genetic aspects. I. Title. II. Series.
[DNLM: 1. Melanoma--etiology. 2. Melanocytes--metabolism.
3. Gene Expression.   QZ 200 H549m 1993]
RC280.M37H474 1993
616.99'47707--dc20
DNlM/DLC
for Library of Congress
93-10991

CONTENTS

LIST OF ABBREVIATIONS

bFGF ....basic factor fibroblast growth factor
BMZ...............basement membrane zone
CAM ....cell adhesion molecule
cAMP ....cyclin adenosine 3',5' monophosphate
CMM ....cutaneous malignant melanoma
DMBA...........demethylbenz[a]anthracene

ECGF ....endothelial cell growth factor
EGF...............epidermal growth factor
GAP ....GTPase activating protein

HB-GAM ....heparin-binding growth associated molecule

HBNF ....heparin-binding neurotrophic factor

HGF ....hepatocyte growth factor
HMWMAA ....high molecular weight melanoma-associated antigen
IGF.................insulin-like growth factor
IL...................interleukin
MAb ....monoclonal antibody
MARCKS ....myristoylated alanine-rich C kinase substrate
MGF...............mast cell growth factor

MGSA ....melanocyte growth stimulatory activity
MHC ....major histocompatibility complex

MIA................melanoma-inhibitory activity
NGF ....nerve growth factor
PDBu 20-Oxo-phorbol-12-13-dibutyrate
PDGF ....platelet-derived growth factor
PK-C ....protein kinase C
PMA..............phorbol 12-myristate-13-acetate
PND...............Pronatriodilatin
RGP ....radial growth phase
SCF.................stem cell growth factor
SF ....scatter factor
TGF...............transforming growth factor
TNF ....tumor necrosis factor
TPA...............12-0-tetradecanoyl-phorbol-13-acetate
UV ....ultraviolet
VEGF ....vascular endothelial cell growth factor
VGP ....vertical growth phase

=CHAPTER 1=

INTRODUCTION

Malignant melanoma is one of the most intensely investigated human malignancies. This wide interest in melanoma research by clinical and experimental investigators has developed for several reasons: 1) the steady increase of melanoma incidence over the past 40 years; 2) the easy accessibility of cutaneous nevi and melanomas for clinical, pathological, and experimental investigations; 3) the relatively high success rate of culturing melanoma cells for experimental studies; and 4) the resistance of advanced melanomas to conventional chemo- and radiation therapy, resulting in a continuously high mortality rate. These factors have also spurred interest in novel therapies such as active or passive immunotherapy, therapies with cytokines or other biological modifiers, or, very recently, gene therapy. Although these new therapeutic modalities show promise for future directions in melanoma treatment, they have not yet resulted in a major impact on reducing disease mortality. This monograph will omit discussions on treatment of melanoma patients, since the various therapies have recently been reviewed.[1] Immunological aspects of melanoma investigations, i.e., the recognition of antigens by patients' antibodies and T cells, and melanoma immune surveillance in patients will also not be discussed. Very recent advances in the identification of antigens inducing a T cell response in melanoma patients[2] and the production of combinatorial (monoclonal) antibodies from human lymphocyte libraries that are displayed on filamentous phages[3-5] suggest that the melanoma immunology field will advance rapidly within the next few years. Current information on immunological approaches in melanoma has been summarized.[6,7]

Several important questions related to the molecular and cellular biology of melanoma cannot yet be addressed due to the lack of experimental data. For example, information is lacking on the transcriptional regulation of tumor growth by oncogenes and suppressor genes. It has also not been possible to address questions regarding the mechanisms of multidrug resistance in melanoma.

Major advances in melanoma research have been made regarding 1) delineation of the different steps of tumor progression using clinical and histopathological criteria,[8,9] 2) culture not only of metastatic melanoma cells but also of primary melanoma cells, nevus cells and normal melanocytes, allowing the biological characterization of cells isolated from different stages of tumor progression [reviewed in ref.10,11] 3) identification of cell surface molecules on melanoma cells with monoclonal antibodies (MAb) [reviewed in ref. 12], which has led to the characterization of melanoma-associated antigen structure and function [reviewed ref. in 13]; 4) characterization of growth factors, cytokines and other biologically active products secreted by melanoma cells that are involved in autocrine and paracrine growth regulation as well as in regulation of invasion and metastasis;[14,15] and 5) identification of chromosome regions that contain melanoma susceptibility genes,[16,17] which may lead to the identification of genes involved in melanoma development and progression.

REFERENCES

1. Balch CM, Houghton AN, Milton GW, Sober AJ, Soong S-J, eds., 2nd edition. Cutaneous melanoma. Philadelphia: J.B. Lippincott Company, 1992.

2. van der Bruggen P, Traversari C, Chomez P, Lurquin C, De Plaen E, Eynde VD, Knuth A, Boon T. A gene encoding an antigen recognized by cytolytic T lymphocytes on a human melanoma. Science 1991; 254:1643-1647.

3. Kasai Y, Herlyn D, Sperlagh M, Maruyama H, Matsushita S, Linnenbach AJ. Molecular cloning of murine monoclonal antiidiotypic Fab. J Immunol Meth 1992; 155:77-89.

4. Kang AS, Barbas CF III, Janda KD, Benkovic SJ, Lerner RA. Linkage of recognition and replication functions by assembling combinatorial antibody Fab libraries along phage surfaces. Proc Natl Acad Sci USA 1991; 88:4363-4366.

5. Barbas CF III, Kang AS, Lerner RA, Benkovic SJ. Assembly of combinatorial antibody libraries on phage surfaces: The gene III site. Proc Natl Acad Sci USA 1991; 88:7978-7982.

6. Hershey P, ed. Biological agents in the treatment of melanoma and other cancers. Proceedings of the International Conference, New Castle, Australia, Sept. 4-7, 1990.

7. Lotze M. Introduction to 1992 Keystone Symposium on "Melanoma and biology of the neural crest". J Immunoth 1992; 12:153.

8. Clark WH Jr, Elder DE, Guerry D IV, Epstein MN, Greene MH, Van Horn M. A study of tumor progression: The precursor lesions of superficial spreading and nodular melanoma. Hum Pathol 1984; 15:1147-1165.

9. Clark WH Jr. Tumour progression and the nature of cancer. Br J Cancer 1991; 64:631-644.

10. Herlyn M. Human melanoma: Development and progression. Cancer Metastasis Rev 1990; 9:101-112.

11. Herlyn M, Kath R, Williams N, Valyi-Nagy I, Rodeck U. Growth regulatory factors for normal, premalignant, and malignant human cells. Adv Cancer Res 1990; 54:213-234.

12. Herlyn M, Koprowski H. Melanoma antigens: Immunological and biological characterization and clinical significance. Ann Rev Immunol 1988; 6:283-308.

13. Herlyn M, Menrad A, Koprowski H. Structure, function and clinical significance of human tumor antigens. J Natl Cancer Inst 1990; 82:1883-1889.

14. Rodeck U, Herlyn M. Growth factors in melanoma. Cancer Metastasis Rev 1991; 10:89-101.

15. Herlyn M, Malkowicz SB. Regulatory pathways in tumor growth and invasion. Lab Invest 1991; 65:262-271.

16. Fountain JW, Karayiorgou M, Ernstoff MS, Kirkwood JM, Vlock DR, Titus-Ernstoff L, Bouchard B, Vihayasaradhi S, Houghton AN, Lahti J, Kidd VJ, Housman DE, Dracopoli NC. Homozygous deletions within chromosome band 9p21 in melanoma. Proc Natl Acad Sci USA 1992; 89:10557-10561.

17. Cannon-Albright LA, Goldgar DE, Meyer LJ, Lewis CM, Anderson DE, Fountain JW, Hegi ME, Wiseman RW, Petty EM, Bale AE, Olufumilayo IO, Diaz MO, Kwiatkowski DJ, Piepkorn MW, Zone JJ, Skolnick MH. Assignment of a locus for familial melanoma, MLM, to chromosome 9p 13-p22. Science 1992; 258:1148-1152.

CHAPTER 2

INCIDENCE OF MELANOMA

The global incidence of melanoma is increasing dramatically,[1-4] and at a faster rate than any other cancer in the United States, Australia, northern Europe, and Canada with the exception of lung cancer in women. In the United States the number of persons with melanoma nearly doubled between 1980 and 1990 (Fig. 1).

Of 32,000 new cases of melanoma diagnosed in 1991, 17,000 occurred in males and 15,000 in females. Approximately 50% of melanomas occur in individuals less than 55 years old. The incidence within individual states in the United States was highest among whites of Hawaii, with 22.7 melanoma cases per 100,000 for men and 18.8 per 100,000 for women. Outside the

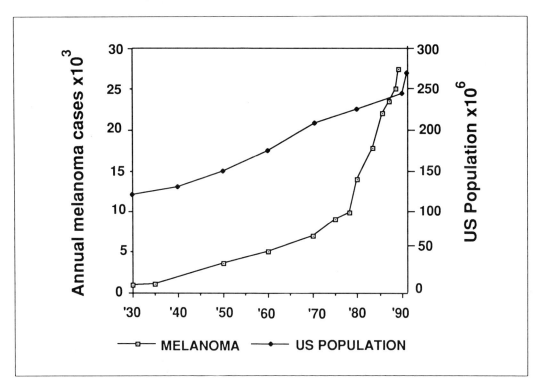

Fig. 1. Comparison of United States population and number of melanoma cases; ◆-◆, US population; ☐-☐, melanoma incidence [adapted from ref. 1].

United States, melanoma incidence has been increasing similarly for the last decades. Most affected countries were New Zealand with rates of 21.4 for women and 15.6 for men per 100,000 individuals, Australia and Norway with 16 and up to 10.5 per 100,000 for males, respectively, and up to 8.9 for females. Other European countries have slightly lower rates. Fortunately, the rising incidence rate exceeds the mortality rate (Fig. 2). The rising gap between incidence and mortality rates suggests that improved early diagnosis and more successful treatment protocols have succeeded in slowing the mortality of melanoma, which was 6,800 in the United States for 1991.[5,6]

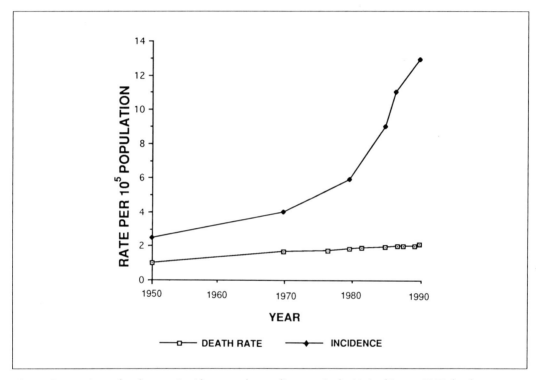

Fig. 2. Comparison of melanoma incidence and mortality rates in the United States, □-□ death rate; ◆-◆, melanoma incidence [adapted from ref. 1].

REFERENCES

1. Grin-Jorgensen CM, Rigel DS, Friedman RJ. The worldwide incidence of malignant melanoma. In: Balch CM, Houghton AN, Milton GW, Sober AJ, Soong S-J, eds. Cutaneous melanoma. Philadelphia: J.B. Lippincott Company, 1992: 27-39.

2. Swerdlow AJ. International trends in cutaneous melanoma. Ann NY Acad Sci 1990; 609:235-251.

3. Lee JA. Trends in melanoma incidence and mortality. Clin Dermatol 1992; 10:9-13.

4. Rigel DS. Epidemiology and prognostic factors in malignant melanoma. Ann Plas Surg 1992; 28:7-8.

5. Roush GC, McCay L, Holford TR. A reversal in the long-term increase in deaths attributable to malignant melanoma. Cancer 1992; 69:1714-1720.

6. Scotto J, Pitcher H, Lee JA. Indications of future decreasing trends in skin-melanoma mortality among whites in the United States. Int J Cancer 1991; 49:490-497.

=========CHAPTER 3=========

ETIOLOGY OF MELANOMA

The etiologic factors leading to the development of melanoma are unknown. However, three major factors are to be considered. First, whites worldwide have a much higher incidence of melanoma than other races and it is 10-fold higher in whites than in blacks. Thus, a negative correlation appears to exist between the degree of skin pigmentation and melanoma on exposed sites.[1] Second, epidemiological and clinical studies point to a role for sunlight in the development of melanoma.[2] However, unlike squamous and basal cell carcinoma of the skin, there is no experimental evidence in humans for a direct causative relation between sunlight exposure and melanoma development in humans. Third, melanoma can be hereditary. Genetic susceptibility for melanoma was first described in 1978 by Clark and Greene for two families.[3] This early observation of an association of cutaneous melanomas with clinically atypical skin moles (dysplastic nevi) segregating in an autosomal fashion has been confirmed by several other groups. Today, familial melanoma accounts for 5 to 10% of all melanoma cases.[4] Individuals with large numbers of nevi have a higher incidence of melanoma than those with low nevus counts,[5] suggesting that in the former, melanocytes have a higher susceptibility for transformation.

THE POTENTIAL ROLE OF ULTRAVIOLET (UV) LIGHT IN MELANOMA DEVELOPMENT

Human melanocytes in the epidermis and nevi and primary melanomas in the epidermis and dermis are exposed to UV light present in sun light, in which UV-B (290-320 nm wave length) is the biologically most active component. UV irradiation can produce multiple alterations in the skin and can induce or exacerbate skin diseases [reviewed in ref. 6-8]. UV irradiation has been found to 1) increase genetic instability by damaging tumor DNA;[9,10] 2) inhibit the endogenous anti-oxidant system;[11,12] 3) alter proto-oncogene and tumor suppressor gene expression;[13] 4) act as a growth factor or growth factor modulator;[14] and 5) suppress cell-mediated immune responses.[15-19] Careful case control studies demonstrate that intermittent high exposure to sunlight during childhood leads to significantly higher incidence of melanoma in adults.[5,20] Not only frequency but also the severity of sunburns appears to determine melanoma development.

Since most experimental studies involving UV irradiation of skin cells were done with keratinocytes, little is known about its contribution to melanoma development. One possible mechanism is the disturbed growth factor network in UV-irradiated human skin. In vitro studies reveal that UV irradiation induces the expression of TGF-α by melanocytes,[21] synthesis of bFGF, IL-1, IL-6 and TNF-α in keratinocytes,[22-25] production of IGF-I by keratinocytes and Langerhans cells,[26] expression of NGF receptor on melanocytes,[27] and increased activity of the melanotropin receptors on melanoma cells.[28] These findings suggest that both normal melanocytes and melanoma cells from early primary lesions can be direct or indirect targets for UV irradiation. Of suppressor genes and oncogenes, p53 mutations have been implicated in 58% of invasive squamous carcinoma of the skin.[29] Activation of the N-*ras* proto-oncogene by an AT to TA or CG transversion at the third position of codon 61 was found in a melanoma cell line from a patient with Xeroderma pigmentosum.[30] This mutation occurred at a dipyrimidine site and is likely initiated by a UV-induced pyrimidine dimer. More recent systematic analyses, however, do not point to major roles for *ras* proto-oncogenes in skin cancer development.[31]

In three experimental animal systems, UV irradiation either causes melanoma or contributes to it. First, Ley and co-workers[32,33] used the South American opossum, *Monodelphis domestica,* as a model because these animals lack a DNA repair mechanism in which UV irradiation-induced pyrimidine dimers are split on the same DNA strand, thus restoring DNA to its original structure. After 70 weeks of UV irradiation, 25% of opossums developed melanocytic tumors, some of which were metastatic. The second model relies on the coadministration of UV irradiation and a chemical carcinogen to newborn C3H mice.[34] In this model, 4-day-old mice received 7,12-dimethylbenz[a]anthracene (DMBA) followed twice weekly by application of croton oil. Addition of UV light dramatically increased time and rate of incidence of melanoma. Combined treatment of UV (UV-A and UV-B) irradiation with DMBA also produced melanomas in hairless mice.[35] Pre-cursor nevus-like lesions and the melanoma samples showed mutations in codon 61 of the N-*ras* gene. The third animal model involves crosses between platyfish and swordtail fish.[36] The fish, after multiple exposures to UV-B, showed a tumor incidence of 20% to 40%.

These experimental models will provide interesting information on the role of UV in melanoma development. Whether this information will also be of value for studies on the etiology of human melanoma remains to be demonstrated.

MOLECULAR GENETICS OF MELANOMA

Various groups have attempted to identify the genetic locus or loci for a dominant melanoma/dysplastic nevus trait. Several regions of the genome have been suggested—through linkage analysis, cytogenetic studies, and identification of loss of heterozygosity—as containing genes associated with dysplastic nevi/melanomas. Studies on genetic abnormalities have focused on chromosomes 1, 6, 7, 9, and 10 because non-random changes have been found on these chromosomes.[37] Melanoma cells are difficult to analyze karyotypically because cells from primary and metastatic lesions show many and often complex abnormalities making it difficult to identify specific nonrandom changes. Figure 3 shows examples of abnormalities which can be defined as deletions, amplifications or rearrangements in primary and metastatic melanomas from the same patients.[38] These studies also point to progression in melanoma as clonal evolution because individual patients show identical abnormalities between early and late lesions. However, final proof of clonal progression of melanoma will come from studies with tissues because cultured cells may have undergone selections. With increased progression, abnormalities increase[39] and these appear to correlate inversely with clinical outcome of the disease,[40] i.e., the more abnormalities, the lower the survival.

CHROMOSOME 1

Linkage analysis studies initially focused on chromosome 1 and, more recently, on chromosome 9, whereas studies on loss of heterozygosity have focused on chromosomes 1 and 6, with scattered findings in other chromosomes. Bale et al[41] found linkage to the rhesus locus and several other markers on chromosome 1p. Later, the same group localized the putative dysplastic nevus/melanoma gene to a region between the anonymous DNA marker D1547 and the gene for pronatriodilatin (PND), 36cM telomeric to the rhesus locus.[42] Several other groups[43-48] have since published seemingly conflicting results. However, these groups did not adhere to the same diagnostic criteria or design as the original study.[42] In a set of Dutch families,[43,44] samples were included from young family members and the criteria for dysplastic nevi were not defined. In the first Utah study,[45] cytologic atypia was not included as a criterion for histologic dysplasia. A more recent re-evaluation of the Utah kindreds[46] considering mole density contradicted earlier results and did

suggest linkage to both D1S47 and PND. In Australia, Kefford et al[47] studied eight kindreds with familial melanoma, but only two of these also had dysplastic nevi in more than two family members. Although those authors reported absence of genetic linkage to chromosome 1p, a small positive lod score at D1S19 was detected when melanoma and dysplastic nevi were analyzed together. They suggest a linkage model for melanoma alone and have refined parameters for the Australian population for age of onset, frequency of sporadic melanomas, incomplete penetrance, and gene frequency. Recently, Nancarrow et al[48] also studied familial melanoma in Australia by linkage analysis. Again most of those families did not have associated dysplastic nevi. Both the Bale and Kefford sets of parameters were used and linkage was excluded to the entire 1p36 region. Very recently, Tucker and co-workers[49] confirmed their initial study,[42] except that heterogeneity was now

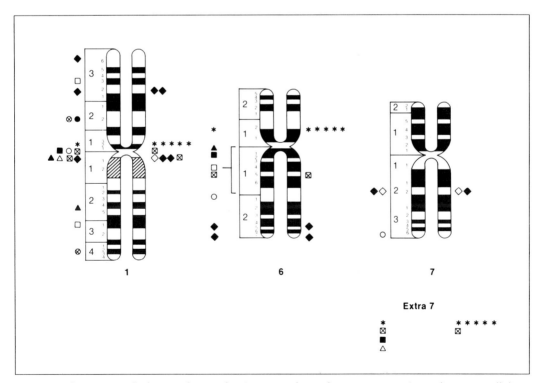

Fig. 3. Chromosomal abnormalities of primary and autologous metastatic melanoma cell lines involving chromosomes #1 (left), #6 (middle), and #7 (right). Sites of chromosomal breakpoints for primary melanoma cell lines are given on the left and for autologous metastatic melanoma cell lines, on the right of each chromosome. Primary and metastatic cell lines of the same patients have the same symbol [adapted from ref. 2].

observed between families, and only a subset of familial melanoma now appears linked to chromosome 1p.

Non-random karyotypic changes involving chromosome 1 have been observed in 53 of 58 advanced melanomas.[50] In most cases, the abnormality was a deletion or translocation of the 1p12-22 region. This region is more proximal than the region implicated in the linkage studies of Bale et al[42] at 1p36. Other malignancies, including neuroblastoma, medullary thyroid carcinoma, pheochromocytoma, and ductal cell carcinoma are also associated with loss of heterozygosity of 1p [summarized in ref. 51]. Three additional cases of advanced melanoma also showed t(1;19)(q23;p13) karyotypes.[52] Dracopoli et al[53] noted that there was frequently loss of heterozygosity of chromosome 1p36 in melanoma, but as a late event in tumor progression. Loss of heterozygosity was found in 43% of 35 melanomas and 52% of 21 melanoma cell lines. The conclusion that the involvement of 1p is a late event in tumor progression came from analysis of multiple metastases derived from the same patient and of melanoma and lymphoblastoid samples from a family with hereditary melanoma.

It cannot be excluded that loss of heterozygosity is an artifact of in vitro culture although Dracopoli et al[53] have shown that loss of heterozygosity genotypes are identical between early and late passages of melanoma cell lines. We have also detected few karyotypic changes during culture,[54] whereas others concluded that several chromosomes, specifically 8, 11, 16, 19, 20, and 22, have the potential to undergo secondary changes in vitro.[55-57]

CHROMOSOME 6

Trent et al[58] noted non-random deletions of 6q in human melanoma cell lines. The subsequent introduction of normal segments of 6q into melanoma cell lines with this deletion suppressed the neoplastic phenotype. 6q also contains the c-*myb* and c-*ras* oncogenes, but in the vast majority of melanocytic tumors studied, there is no evidence that these are abnormally expressed.[59] However, a loss of heterozygosity for loci in 6q22-q23 and 6q24-q27 in melanoma metastases was recently reported.[24]

CHROMOSOME 7

An experimental model of melanoma in the swordtail/platyfish implicates two genes, including a tumor suppressor gene, *Tu*, as responsible for the tumor phenotype.[61] *Tu* encodes a receptor tyrosine kinase homologous to the human EGF receptor, which maps to the 7p11-13 region frequently rearranged in melanoma.[39] Expression of the EGF receptor on human melanoma cells correlates with increased dosage of chromosome 7.[62]

CHROMOSOME 9

Chromosome 9 has been increasingly analyzed for the presence of a putative melanoma susceptibility gene. Suggestive evidence comes from several groups: a) Fountain et al[63] detected a 2-3 megabase region proximal to the interferon-α gene cluster (9p21-p22) that is heterozygously or homozygously deleted in 85% of melanoma tumor and cell line DNAs; b) Petty et al[64] reported a constitutional cytogenetic abnormality associated with sporadic cutaneous malignant melanoma/dysplastic nevus syndrome, i.e., a *de novo* unbalanced translocation: 46, XX, -5, -9, + der(5) t(5;9)(p13.3;p13.3). Parmiter et al[65] also noted a dysplastic nevus syndrome patient, who had a t(9;10)(q24;q24) karyotype in one of the excised nevi.

Two groups have assigned a locus for a familial melanoma susceptibility gene to chromosome 9p13-p22, a 2-4 megabase region between the loci for the interferon-α gene and the marker D9S3. In the majority of melanomas (12 out of 14) studied by Fountain et al,[66] this region was either deleted or rearranged in one of the two copies. Furthermore, in 10% of the melanoma cell lines, another marker, D9S126, which resides between the two, was deleted from both copies of chromosome 9. Such disarray strongly suggests a role for this stretch of DNA in the progression of melanoma, although the possibility that changes occur after cancer development cannot be ruled out. The work of Skolnick and co-workers[67] also showed that a region flanked by the interferon-α gene and the D9S126 marker contains a gene predisposing to human melanoma. That study relied only on melanoma as a diagnostic criterion and not on the diagnosis of dysplastic nevi. It involved 11 extended kindreds with 82 cases of melanoma and a single family with 53 members, 22 of whom had melanoma. Support for a melanoma predisposition gene on chromosome 9p came from identification of a 34-year-old Caucasian woman with multiple atypical nevi and eight primary cutaneous melanomas who had a germline cytogenetic rearrangement involving chromosomes 5p and 9p. Molecular analyses revealed loss of material from the 9p21 region. The interferon-α and D9S126 loci from this individual were compared to those of her unaffected parents; gene dosage studies showed homozygosity at both loci, suggesting that the germline loss of this region predisposes to melanoma.[68] The 9p linkage analyses also suggest genetic heterogeneity because of the findings from kindreds who are affected with melanoma but do not show the deletions.

Chromosome 10

Parmiter et al[65] reported multiple alterations of chromosome 10q in association with early stages of melanocytic neoplasia. One of 10 dysplastic nevi had the t(9;10)(p24;q24) translocation noted above. Out of three complex primary melanomas studied, one showed a loss of chromosome 10 and another had a t(10?)(q26;?). In 51 advanced melanomas (both primary and metastatic), 18 had lost one or more copies of chromosome 10 and one other had a complex three-way rearrangement: 46, XY, t(5, 6, 10) with breakpoints on chromosome 10 at q23 and q25.[69] These data suggest that 10q may also harbor a locus for a gene or genes involved in early stages of melanoma development.

ONCOGENES AND SUPPRESSOR GENES

c-ras

Several studies have addressed the question of *ras* proto-oncogene activation in hu-

man malignant melanomas. The oncogenes H-*ras*, K-*ras*, and N-*ras* encode similar proteins with molecular weights of 21,000 (p21). *Ras* oncogenes are closely related to the family of membrane-bound guanine nucleotide-binding proteins, the G proteins, which are activated in response to extracellular signals and play an important role in the regulation of second messengers. Mutational analysis of *ras* oncoproteins revealed amino acid alterations at codons 12, 13 and 61, which resulted in constitutive activation of these mutant *ras*-encoded proteins and, in turn, uncontrolled second-messenger production.[70,71] Expression of all three *ras* oncogenes has been detected in melanoma cells.[72-75] Upon transfection of melanoma DNAs into NIH3T3 cells, activated N-*ras* and H-*ras* genes were detected in 4 of 30 different melanomas tested.[72] Albino et al[76] found N-*ras* and H-*ras* mutations at codon 61 in about 24% of cultured melanoma cells. Those metastatic melanoma cells expressing mutated N-*ras* and H-*ras* had a very similar phenotype, characterized by high expression of EGF receptor and class II histocompatibility antigens, lack of pigmentation, and an epithelioid spindle-type morphology.[76] Noncultured melanomas had the mutated *ras* genes in 5 to 6% of the specimens. Interestingly, *ras* gene expression was not detected in specimens from normal and dysplastic nevi.[76] We have detected activated N-*ras* genes in 3 of 19 (16%) metastatic melanomas analyzed, but in none of 6 VGP primary melanomas tested.[77] Activation of N-*ras* genes, indicated by the presence of an 8.8 kb fragment, was found in secondary NIH3T3 transformants derived from three separate metastases of the same patient. In another study, N-*ras* mutations were detected exclusively in tumor samples obtained from sun-exposed locations of the body, suggesting a close correlation between UV irradiation and this type of *ras* mutation.[78] In contrast to the results in the former studies, Shukla et al[79] detected mutations of the K-*ras* gene at codon 12 in 20% of the genomic DNA samples examined from melanoma specimens. Moreover, these mutations were also found in benign nevi and primary melanomas, suggesting the importance of *ras* activation even during melanoma development. Another transforming gene, c-*mel* which is weakly related to the *ras* gene, has been found in a melanoma cell line.[80,81]

Although mutated *ras* oncogenes have reportedly clear effects on normal diploid melanocytes, including changes in their growth characteristics,[82,83] and *ras* represents the family of oncogenes most consistently and frequently expressed in human malignant melanomas, their biological function remains to be determined. Genes of the *ras* family represent possible candidates for the role of regulators of cytokine expression in human tumors. H-*ras* mutation can influence expression of cytokines in fibroblasts.[84] In melanoma, mutations of N-*ras* correlate with expression IL-1α, IL-6, and TNF-α genes (G. Parmiani, personal communication).

c-src

An association between the c-*src* proto-oncogene, a nonreceptor membrane-associated tyrosine kinase, and melanoma development is unclear. Elevated levels of pp60[c-src] kinase were detected in cell extracts of human melanomas,[85] but a comparison between normal melanocytes and melanoma cell lines did not reveal differences in the level or size of c-*src* transcripts.[82] Others have found more extensive phosphorylation of *src* at the tyrosine 530 position in melanomas than in melanocytes.[86]

c-myb

Alterations of nuclear proto-oncogenes have been reported for the c-*myb* oncogene. In 1 of 30 analyzed melanoma cell lines, Linnenbach et al[87] found rearrangements of c-*myb* in connection with a 6q22 chromosomal abnormality. Further analysis revealed that this rearrangement leads to a deletion in the 3'-end of the c-*myb* locus and concomitant translocation of a portion of chromosome 12 to chromosome 6.[88] Although Trent and co-workers[89] did not detect any rearrangement of the *myb* gene, they did find alterations in band 6q13, the region for the *myb* gene.

c-myc

Melanoma cells frequently show increased expression of the *c-myc* proto-oncogene,[91,92]

Table 1. Oncogenes and suppressor genes implicated in melanoma development

Gene	Procedure for detection	Comments	Reference
n-ras	NIH3T3 transformation	5-20% frequency	72,116
myb	Gene rearrangement	<5% frequency	87,88
myc	Overexpression	50% frequency	90
ret	Transgenic mice	Hyperpigmentation	94
nm23	Subtraction hybridization	Suppressed in metastasis	97
E1A	Transfection	Growth suppression	100
p53	Mutations	10-40% frequency	116,117
kit	Suppression of expression	60% frequency	130-132
tu/mrk	Fish breeding	Oncogene/suppressor gene cooperation	102,103
NF1	Deletion	2 of 8 cell lines	141

but overexpression was mostly found only in high-passage cell lines, suggesting the possibility of culture artifacts.[91] The relative abundance of c-*myc* is generally associated with tumorigenicity parameters such as anchorage-independent growth in soft agar and ability to transform NIH3T3 cells in transfection assays.

Overexpression of c-*myc* in melanomas correlates with downregulation of HLA-B in these cells,[90] suggesting that they are less likely to be immunologically recognized. Thus, c-*myc* might contribute indirectly to tumor progression. However, more recent investigations could not confirm c-*myc* overexpression with HLA-B downregulation (F. Marincola, personal communication). Amplification of the N-*myc* gene was also found in the melanoma tissues of two patients; the patient with four extra copies of n-*myc* relapsed after initial therapy earlier than the patient with one extra copy of n-*myc*,[93] but it remains to be shown whether n-*myc* gene amplification correlates with survival in melanoma patients.

c-*ret*

The *ret* proto-oncogene encodes a receptor-type tyrosine kinase and is often expressed in human tumors of neuroectodermal origin such as neuroblastoma, pheochromocytoma, and thyroid medullary carcinoma. Mice transgenic for *ret* showed hyperpigmentation due to aberrant melanogenesis and melanoma development.[94] Established cell lines from these tumors were highly invasive and metastatic when transplanted to athymic nude mice.[95]

c-*fos* and c-*jun*

In normal melanocytes, expression of c-*fos* and c-*jun* depended on the growth-promoting factors in medium, whereas in melanomas, both were activated irrespective of culture growth conditions.[96] In low expressing melanoma cells, c-*fos* and c-*jun* expression was inducible with serum if the cells were dependent on exogenous growth factors.

nm23

The *nm23* gene, originally identified by differential hybridization experiments involving murine K-1735 melanoma sublines with either low or high metastatic potential, may function as a metastasis suppressor.[97] Expression of *nm23* gene inversely correlates with tumor progression. Melanoma patients developing metastases during the first two years after diagnosis had significantly lower levels of tumor *nm23* expression compared to patients with less aggressive disease.[98] When highly metastatic K-1733 melanoma cells were transfected with the *nm23-1* gene, cells showed reduced metastatic potential and altered responses to growth factors.[99]

E1A

Stable expression of the adenovirus 5 *E1A* gene in human melanoma cells reduced anchorage-independent growth and tumorigenic potential, caused cytoskeletal reorganization, induced flat morphology, and restored contact inhibition.[100] By these criteria, *E1A* appears functionally to be a tumor suppressor gene. The apparent paradox arising from the observation that *E1A* transforms rodent cells in cooperation with other oncogenes suggests that it may be the prototype of a class of growth regulatory proteins having both transforming and anti-oncogenic activities in specific context.

Tu/Xmrk

Two fish of the genus *Xiphophorus*, the platyfish (*X. maculatus*) and the swordtail (*X. helleri*) provide a genetic model for identifying melanoma oncogenes and suppressor genes. Malignant melanomas form only in the F1 progeny between platyfish carrying the dominant tumor formation gene (*Tu*) with *X. helleri* if the repressor gene R is absent [reviewed in ref. 101]. The *Tu* gene encodes *Xmrk*, a membrane receptor tyrosine kinase that is similar but not identical to the EGF receptor.[102] A 4.7 kb transcript is expressed in the melanomas of fish with the *Tu* gene and is found at low levels in benign and at high levels in malignant lesions. The R gene and the *Tu/Xmrk* gene apparently cooperate.[103] The 5' fragment of *Xmrk* is a strong promoter in melanoma cells that do not carry the R locus. This fragment is also present in a separate locus (D) found in all *Xiphophorus* cells, suggesting that the *Tu* locus arose by non-homologous recombination of the *Xmrk* proto-oncogene and the D locus. The recombined form of *Xmrk* is present in all *Xiphophorus* with the *Tu* locus. Thus, the control of melanomas by the repressor locus can be viewed as an incidental side-effect of the regulation exerted by the R gene on the D locus.[103]

p53

The p53 gene on chromosome 17p13.1 encodes a nuclear protein, which is implicated in cell proliferation and tumor progression. Whereas the wild-type form has tumor suppressor properties, various mutations inactivate these capabilities.[104,105] There is increasing evidence that mutations in the p53 gene are among the most common somatic genetic alterations in human cancer.[105] Loss of wild-type p53 protein and expression of mutant forms have been demonstrated in a high proportion of malignant tumors of colon,[106,107] breast[108-110] and brain, and, at lower frequencies, in cancers of the liver, bladder, esophagus and head and neck as well as sarcomas.[105,111] Germline mutations of the locus are also predisposing to Li-Fraumeni syndrome, a heritable cancer syndrome.[112]

A high frequency of mutations in the p53 gene has been reported in skin cancer of both squamous cell[113] and basal cell[114] skin carcinomas. To date, only few analyses of p53 alterations in cutaneous malignant melanomas have been reported. In one study overexpression of p53 protein was detected by indirect immunofluorescence in more than 80% of the malignant melanomas examined.[115] In another, however, a p53 gene mutation and overexpression of p53 protein was found in only 1 of 9 melanoma cell lines.[116] Weiss et al[117] detected p53 mutations in 4 of 13 cell lines tested; 3 of these mutations were C to T transversions. Such alterations might reflect

UV-induced damage, because they have also been found in basal and squamous cell carcinomas of the skin[113,114] and UV-light has been shown to induce specific mutation.[118]

c-*kit*

The proto-oncogene c-*kit* is the cellular homolog of v-*kit*, the oncogene of an acute transforming feline retrovirus.[119] c-*kit* is a transmembrane receptor tyrosine kinase. In the mouse, c-*kit* maps to the dominant white spotting locus (*W*). Mutations of this locus affect various aspects of hematopoiesis and also migration of melanoblasts during development; white spotting results from a partial failure of melanocytes to populate the skin due to mutations in c-*kit*.[120-128] A mutation in the tyrosine kinase domain of c-*kit*, which results in substitution of glycine with arginine at codon 664, was found in patients with autosomal dominant piebaldism.[129,130]

Expression of c-*kit* in human melanomas is reduced when compared to expression on normal melanocytes.[131-133] Suppression of c-*kit* expression has also been observed in mouse melanomas.[122] Point mutations affecting the catalytic region in the kinase domain of the *kit* protein appears to lead to a growth disadvantage of melanocytes which may, in turn, allow selection of melanocytes that mobilize more efficient metabolic pathways.[134] These conclusions were drawn from observations in Wf/Wf mutant mice, in which most isolated melanocytes did not proliferate, but a few surviving cells spontaneously transformed and became invasive melanomas. Studies from mouse melanocyte cell lines with mutations at the silver and recessive spotting loci, which map close to the c-*kit* locus, raise the possibility that additional loci in the same region of mouse chromosome 5 regulate melanocyte proliferation and immortality.[135]

nck

nck cDNA was originally isolated in melanoma with a MAb to the MUC18 antigen.[136] This cDNA encodes a protein of 377 amino acids which lacks a signal peptide or transmembrane region. *nck* does not show homology with MUC18, but consists of one SH2 (*src* homology) and three SH3 domains. The *src* homology motif of the *nck* gene is found in nonreceptor tyrosine kinases, *ras* GTPase-activating protein (GAP), phosphotidylinositol-3 kinase, and phospholipase C-g. Three laboratories have recently identified the *nck* sequence as a new oncogene.[137-139] Overexpression of human *nck* in rat fibroblasts results in transformation.[137] The *nck* protein is phosphorylated on tyrosine, serine, and threonine residues.[138] Since *nck* is the target for a variety of protein kinases, a role for *nck* as an adaptor for the physical and functional coordination of signalling proteins has been postulated.[139]

NF1

The *NF1* gene maps to chromosome 17 and is deleted in neuroblastoma[140] and melanoma.[141] Homozygous deletion of most of the *NF1* gene in 1 of 8 malignant melanoma cell lines resulted in loss of detectable *NF1* mRNA and protein. Potentially, *NF1* is a recessive tumor suppressor gene[142] whose loss of function appears to be associated with neurofibromatosis and cancer. The *NF1* gene shares homology with the *ras* GTPase activator p120. The GAP-related domain in neurofibronin, the gene product of *NF1*, is capable of downregulating $p21^{ras}$ by stimulating its intrinsic GTPase activity. Thus, neurofibronin may act as a negative regulator of $p21^{ras}$-mediated signal transduction. These very recent findings add another gene to investigations of the molecular genetics of melanoma.

SUMMARY

In summary, several oncogenes and suppressor genes have been implicated in melanoma progression. However, of more than 40 genes tested in various laboratories, none has been shown to be involved in the majority of melanomas studied. With the exception of the cooperation of the R and *Tu* genes in fish melanoma, no gene amplification, mutation, or rearrangement has yet been discovered that could demonstrate sequential changes in cells before or after transformation. Fortunately, this lack of experimental evidence has encouraged additional laboratories to enter the search. The recently discovered role of c-*kit* in melanoblast migration and its downregulation in melanomas has renewed interest in this tyrosine kinase and its role or that of related genes in melanoma formation. Several laboratories have begun to use new technological developments for subtractive isolation of specific RNA of melanoma cells and cloning the corresponding genes. The first reports have provided interesting information on genes whose constitutive activation might contribute to melanoma development.[143,144] Others have identified an activated calcium-binding protein as a correlate of melanoma progression (K. Jimbow, personal communication) or an amplified IGF-I receptor gene (J. Trent, personal communication).

REFERENCES

1. Crombie IK. Racial differences in melanoma incidence. Br J Cancer 1979; 40:185-193.
2. Rigel DS. Epidemiology and prognostic factors in malignant melanoma. Ann Plas Surg 1992; 28:7-8.
3. Clark WH Jr, Reimer RR, Greene M, Ainsworth AM, Mastrangelo MJ. Origin of familial malignant melanomas from heritable melanocytic lesions. Arch Dermatol 1978; 114:732.
4. Greene MH, Fraumeni JF. The hereditary variant of malignant melanoma. In. Clark WH, Goldman L, Mastrangelo MJ, eds. Human malignant melanoma. New York: Grune and Stratton, 1979; pp 139-166,
5. Gallagher RP, McLean DI, Yang CP, Coldman AJ, Silver HK, Spinelli JJ, Beagrie M. Suntan, sunburn, and pigmentation factors and the frequency of acquired melanocytic nevi in children. Similarities to melanoma: The Vancouver mole study. Arch Dermatol 1990; 126:770-776.
6. Matsui MS, DeLeo VA. Longwave ultraviolet radiation and promotion of skin cancer. Cancer Cells 1991; 3:8-12.
7. Longstretch JD, Lea CS, Kripke ML. Ultraviolet radiation and other putative causes of melanoma. In: Balch CM, Houghton AN, Milton GW, Sober AJ, Soong S-J, eds. Cutaneous melanoma. Philadelphia: J.B. Lippincott Company, 1992; pp 46-58.

8. Elwood JM. Melanoma and ultraviolet irradiation. Clin Dermatol 1992; 10:41-50.

9. Cifone MA, Fidler IJ. Increasing metastatic potential is associated with increasing genetic instability of clones isolated from murine neoplasms. Proc Natl Acad Sci USA 1981; 78:6949-6952.

10. Megidish T, Mazurek N. A mutant protein kinase C that can transform fibroblasts. Nature 1989; 342:807-811.

11. Fuchs J, Packer L. Ultraviolet irradiation and the skin antioxidant system. Photodermatol Photoimmunol Photomed 1990; 7:90-92.

12. Rabiloud T, Asselineau D, Miquel C, Calvayrac R, Darmon M, Vuillaume M. Deficiency in catalase activity correlates with the appearance of tumor phenotype in human keratinocytes. Int J Cancer 1990; 45:952-956.

13. Ronai AZ, Okin E, Weinstein IB. Ultraviolet light induces the expression of oncogenes in rat fibroblast and human keratinocytes. Oncogene 1988; 2:201-204.

14. Libow LF, Scheide S, Deleo VA. Ultraviolet radiation acts as an independent mitogen for normal human melanocytes in culture. Pigment Cell Res 1988; 1:397-401.

15. Penn I. Ultraviolet light and skin cancer. Immunol Today 1985; 6:206-207.

16. Noonan FP, DeFabo EC. Ultraviolet B dose-response curves for local and systemic immunosuppression are identical. Photochem Photobiol 1990; 52:801-810.

17. Kripke ML. Ultraviolet radiation and tumor immunity. J Reticuloendothel Soc 1977; 22:217-222.

18. Granstein RD. Photoimmunology. Semin Dermatol 1990; 9:16-24.

19. Donowho CK, Kripke ML. Immunologic factors in melanoma. Clin Dermatol 1992; 10:69-74.

20. Osterlind A, Tucker MA, Stone BJ, Jensen OM. The Danish case-control study of cutaneous malignant melanoma. II. Importance of UV-light exposure. Int J Cancer 1988; 42:319-324.

21. Ellem KAO, Cullinan M, Baumann KC, Dunstan A. UVR induction of TGF-α: A possible autocrine mechanism for the epidermal melanocytic response and for promotion of epidermal carcinogenesis. Carcinogenesis 1988; 9:797-801.

22. Halaban R, Langdon R, Birchall N, Cuono C, Baird A, Scott G, Moellmann G, McGuire J. Basic fibroblast growth factor from human keratinocytes is a natural mitogen for melanocytes. J Cell Biol 1988; 107:1611-1619.

23. Kupper TS, Chua AO, Flood P, McGuire J, Gubler U. Interleukin 1 gene expression in cultured human keratinocytes is augmented by ultraviolet irradiation. J Clin Invest 1987; 80:430-436.

24. Kirnbauer R, Köck A, Neuner P, Förster E, Krutmann J, Urbanski A, Schauer E, Ansel JC, Schwarz T, Luger TA. Regulation of epidermal cell interleukin-6 production by UV light and corticosteroids. J Invest Dermatol 1991; 96:484-489.

25. Köck A, Schwarz T, Kirnbauer R, Urbanski A, Perry P, Ansel JC, Luger TA. Human keratinocytes are a source for tumor necrosis factor a: Evidence for synthesis and release upon stimulation with endotoxin or ultraviolet light. J Exp Med 1990; 172:1609-1614.

26. Hansson H-A, Johnsson R, Petruson K. Transiently increased insulin-like growth factor. I. Immunoreactivity in UVB-irradiated mouse skin. J Invest Dermatol 1988; 91:328-332.

27. Peacocke M, Yaar M, Mansur CP, Chao MV, Gilchrest BA. Induction of nerve growth factor receptors on cultured human melanocytes. Proc Natl Acad Sci USA 1988; 85:5282-5286.

28. Birchall N, Orlow SJ, Kupper T, Pawelek J. Interactions between ultraviolet light and interleukin-1 on MSH binding in both mouse melanoma and human squamous carcinoma cells. Biochem Biophys Res Commun 1991; 175:839-845.

29. Brash DE, Rudolph JA, Simon JA, Lin A, McKenna GJ, Baden HP, Halperin AJ, Pontén J. A role for sunlight in skin cancer: UV-induced p53 mutations in squamous cell carcinoma. Proc Natl Acad Sci USA 1991; 88:10124-10128.

30. Keijzer W, Mulder MP, Langeveld JC, Smit EM, Bos JL, Bootsma D, Hoeijmakers JH. Establishment and characterization of a melanoma cell line from a xeroderma pigmentosum patient: Activation of N-*ras* at a potential pyrimidine dimer site. Cancer Res 1989; 49:1229-1235.

31. Törmänen VT, Pfeifer GP. Mapping of UV photoproducts within *ras* proto-oncogenes in

UV-irradiated cells: Correlation with mutations in human skin cancer. Oncogene 1992; 7:1729-1736.

32. Ley RD. Photoreactivation of UV-induced pyrimidine dimers and erythema in the marsupial *Monodelphis domestica*. Proc Natl Acad Sci USA 1985; 82:2409-2411.

33. Ley RD, Applegate LA, Padilla RS, Stuart TD. Ultraviolet radiation-induced malignant melanoma in *Monodelphis domestica*. Photochem Photobiol 1989; 50:1-5.

34. Romerdahl CA, Stephens LC, Bucana C, Kripke ML. The role of ultraviolet radiation in the induction of melanocytic skin tumors in inbred mice. Cancer Communications 1989; 1:209-216.

35. Husain Z, Pathak MA, Flotte T, Wick MM. Role of ultraviolet radiation in the induction of melanocytic tumors in hairless mice following 7,12-dimethylbenz[a]anthracene application and ultraviolet irradiation. Cancer Res 1991 51:4964-4970.

36. Setlow RB, Woodhead AD, Grist E. Animal model for ultraviolet radiation-induced melanoma: Playtyfish-swordtail hybrid. Proc Natl Acad Sci USA 1989; 86:8922-8926.

37. Trent JM. Cytogenetics of human malignant melanoma. In: Balch CM, Houghton AN, Milton GW, Sober AJ, Soong S-J, eds. Cutaneous melanoma. Philadelphia: J.B. Lippincott Company, 1992; pp 101-111.

38. Kath R, Rodeck U, Parmiter A, Jambrosic J, Herlyn M. Growth factor independence in vitro of primary melanoma cells from advanced but not early or intermediate lesions. Cancer Therapy and Control 1990; 1:179-191.

39. Balaban G, Herlyn M, Guerry D IV, Bartolo R, Koprowski H, Clark WH Jr, Nowell PC. Cytogenetics of human malignant melanoma and premalignant lesions. Cancer Genet Cytogenet 1984; 11:429-439.

40. Trent JM, Meyskens FL, Salmon SE, Ryschon K, Leong SPL, Davis JR, McGee DL. Relation of cytogenetic abnormalities and clinical outcome in metastatic melanoma. N Engl J Med 1990; 322:1508-1511.

41. Bale SJ, Dracopoli NC, Greene MH, Gerhard DS, Housman DE. Linkage analysis of melanoma and dysplastic nevus syndrome with polymorphic loci on human chromosome 1p (abstr). Cytogenet Cell Genet 1987; 46:575A.

42. Bale SJ, Dracopoli NC, Tucker MA, Clark WH Jr, Fraser MC, Stanger BZ, Green P, Donis-Keller H, Housman DE, Greene MH. Mapping the gene for hereditary cutaneous malignant melanoma-dysplastic nevus to chromosome 1p. N Engl J Med 1989; 320:1367-1372.

43. van Haeringen A, Bergman W, Nelen MR, van der Kooij-Meijs E, Hendrikse I, Wijnen JT, Khan PM, Klasen EC, Frants RR. Exclusion of the dysplastic nevus syndrome (DNS) locus from the short arm of chromosome 1 by linkage studies in Dutch families. Genomics 1989; 5:61-64.

44. Gruis NA, Bergman W, Frants RR. Locus for susceptibility to melanoma on chromosome 1p. N Engl J Med 1990; 322:853-854.

45. Cannon-Albright LA, Goldgar DE, Wright EC, Turco A, Jost M, Meyer LJ, Piepkorn M, Zone JJ, Skolnick MH. Evidence against the reported linkage of the cutaneous melanoma-dysplastic nevus syndrome locus to chromosome 1p36. Am J Hum Genet 1990; 46:912-918.

46. Goldgar DE, Cannon-Albright LA, Meyer LJ, Piepkorn MW, Zone JJ, Skolnick MH. Inheritance of nevus number and size in melanoma and dysplastic nevus kindreds. J Natl Cancer Inst 1991; 23:1726-1733.

47. Kefford RF, Salmon J, Shaw HM, Donald JA, McCarthy WH. Hereditary melanoma in Australia: Variable association with dysplastic nevi and absence of genetic linkage to chromosome 1p. Cancer Genet Cytogenet 1991; 51:45-55.

48. Nancarrow DJ, Palmer JM, Walters MK, Kerr BM, Hafner GJ, Garske L, McLeod GR, Hayward NK. Exclusion of the familial melanoma locus (MLM) from the PND/D1S47 and MYCL1 regions of chromosome arm 1p in 7 Australian pedigrees. Genomics 1992; 12:18-25.

49. Goldstein AM, Dracopoli NC, Ho EC, Fraser MC, Kearns KS, Bale SJ, McBride OW, Clark WH Jr, Tucker MA. Further evidence for a locus for cutaneous malignant melanoma-dysplastic nevus (CMM/DN) on chromosome 1p and evidence for genetic heterogeneity. Am J Hum Genet, In press.

50. Parmiter AH, Nowell PC. The cytogenetics of human malignant melanoma and premalignant

lesions. In: Nathanson L, ed. Malignant melanoma: Biology, diagnosis, and therapy. Boston: Kluwer Academic Publishers, 1988:47-61.

51. Weinberg RA. Tumor suppressor genes. Science 1991; 254:1138-1152.

52. Parmiter AH, Balaban G, Herlyn M, Clark WH Jr, Nowell PC. A t(1;19) chromosome translocation in three cases of human malignant melanoma. Cancer Res 1986; 46:1526-1529.

53. Dracopoli NC, Harnett P, Bale SJ, Stanger BZ, Tucker MA, Housman DE, Kefford RF. Loss of alleles from the distal short arm of chromosome 1 occurs late in melanoma tumor progression. Proc Natl Acad Sci USA 1989; 86:4614-4618.

54. Herlyn M, Balaban G, Bennicelli J, Guerry D IV, Halaban R, Herlyn D, Elder DE, Maul GG, Steplewski Z, Nowell PC, Clark WH Jr, Koprowski H. Primary melanoma cells of the vertical growth phase: Similarities to metastatic cells. J Natl Cancer Inst 1985; 74:283-289.

55. Kakati S, Song SY, Sandberg AA. Chromosomes and causation of human cancer and leukemia. XXII. Karyotypic changes in malignant melanoma. Cancer 1977; 40:1173-1181.

56. Atkin NB, Baker MC. A metastatic malignant melanoma with 24 chromosomes. Hum Genet 1981; 58:217-219.

57. Becher R, Gibas Z, Karakousis C, Sandberg AA. Nonrandom chromosome changes in malignant melanoma. Cancer Res 1983; 43:5010-5016.

58. Trent JM, Stanbridge EJ, McBride HL, Meese EU, Casey G, Araujo DE, Witkowski CM, Nagle RB. Tumorigenicity in human melanoma cell lines controlled by introduction of human chromosome 6. Science 1989; 247:568-571.

59. Linnenbach AJ, Huebner K, Reddy EP, Herlyn M, Parmiter AH, Nowell PC, Koprowski H. Structural alteration in the MYB protooncogene and deletion within the gene encoding a-type protein kinase C in human melanoma cell lines. Proc Natl Acad Sci USA 1988; 85:74-78.

60. Millikin D, Meese E, Vogelstein B, Witkowski C, Trent J. Loss of heterozygosity for loci on the long arm of chromosome 6 in human malignant melanoma. Cancer Res 1991; 51:5449-5453.

61. Wittbrodt J, Adam D, Malitscheck B, Mäueler W, Raulf F, Telling A, Robertson SM, Schartl, M. Novel putative receptor tyrosine kinase encoded by the melanoma-inducing *Tu* locus in *Xiphophorus*. Nature 1989; 341:415-421.

62. Koprowski H, Herlyn M, Balaban G, Parmiter A, Ross A, Nowell P. Expression of the receptor for epidermal growth factor correlates with increased dosage of chromosome 7 in malignant melanoma. Somat Cell Mol Genet 1985; 11:297-302.

63. Fountain JW, Karayiorgou M, Graw SL, Buckler AJ, Taruscio D, Ward DC, Ernstoff MS, Kirkwood JM, Andersen LB, Collins FS, Dracopoli NC, Housman DE. Chromosome 9p involvement in melanoma. Am J Hum Genet 1991; 49:A45.

64. Petty EM, Bale AE, Bolognia JL, Yang-Feng TL. A constitutional cytogenetic abnormality associated with cutaneous malignant melanoma/dysplastic nevus syndrome (CMM/DNS). Am J Hum Genet 1991; 49:A247.

65. Parmiter AH, Balaban G, Clark WH Jr, Nowell PC. Possible involvement of the chromosome region 10q24-q26 in early stages of melanocytic neoplasia. Cancer Genet Oncogenet 1988; 30:313-317.

66. Fountain JW, Karayiorgou M, Ernstoff MS, Kirkwood JM, Vlock DR, Titus-Ernstoff L, Bouchard B, Vihayasaradhi S, Houghton AN, Lahti J, Kidd VJ, Housman DE, Dracopoli NC. Homozygous deletions within chromosome band 9p21 in melanoma. Proc Natl Acad Sci USA 1992; 89:10557-10561.

67. Cannon-Albright LA, Goldgar DE, Meyer LJ, Lewis CM, Anderson DE, Fountain JW, Hegi ME, Wiseman RW, Petty EM, Bale AE, Olufunmilayo IO, Diaz MO, Kwiatkowski DJ, Piepkorn MW, Zone JJ, Skolnick MH. Assignment of a locus for familial melanoma, MLM, to chromosome 9p 13-p22. Science 1992; 258:1148-1152.

68. Petty EM. Cited as personal comunication in reference 31.

69. Parmiter AH, Balaban G, Clark WH Jr, Nowell PC. Possible involvement of the chromosome region 10q to q26 in early stages of melanocytic neoplasia. Cancer Genet Cytogenet 1988; 30:313-317.

70. Bos JL. *Ras* oncogene in human cancer: A review. Cancer Res 1989; 49:4682-4689.

71. Hall A. The cellular functions of small GTP-binding proteins. Science 1990; 249:635-640.

72. Albino AP, Le Strange R, Oliff AI, Furth ME, Old LJ. Transforming *ras* genes from human melanoma: A manifestation of tumour heterogeneity? Nature 1984; 308:69-72.

73. Sekiya T, Fushimi M, Hori H, Hirohashi S, Nishimura S, Sugimura T. Molecular cloning and the total nucleotide sequence of the human c-Ha-*ras*-1-gene activated in a melanoma from a Japanese patient. Proc Natl Acad Sci USA 1984; 81:4771-4775.

74. Raybaud F, Nuguchi T, Marics I, Adelaid J, Planche J, Batoz M, Aubert C, de Lapeyriere O, Birnbaum D. Detection of a low frequency of activated *ras* genes in human melanomas using a tumorigenicity assay. Cancer Res 1988; 48:950-953.

75. Padua RA, Barrass NC, Curie GA. Activation of N-*ras* in a human melanoma cell line. Mol Cell Biol 1985; 5:582-585.

76 Albino AP, Nanus DM, Mentle IR, Cordon-Cardo C, McNutt NS, Bressler J, Andreeff M. Analysis of *ras* oncogenes in malignant melanoma and precursor lesions: Correlation of point mutations with differentiation phenotype. Oncogene 1989; 4:1363-1374.

77. Graeven U, Becker D, Herlyn M. Structural and functional characteristics of human melanoma. In: Pretlow, TG, Pretlow, TP, eds. Biochemical and molecular aspects of selected cancers, Vol. 1. Orlando: Academic Press, 1991; pp 151-176.

78. Van't Veer LJ, Burgering BMT, Versteet R, Boot AJM, Ruiter DJ, Osanto S, Schrier PI, Bos JL. N-*ras* mutations in human cutaneous melanoma from sun-exposed body sites. Mol Cell Biol 1989; 9:3114-3116.

79. Shukla VK, Hughes DC, McCormick F, Padua RA. *Ras* mutations in human melanotic lesions: K-*ras* activation is a frequent and early event in melanoma development. Oncogene Res 1989; 5:121-127.

80. Padua R, Barrass N, Currie GA. A novel transforming gene in a human malignant melanoma cell line. Nature 1984; 311:671-673.

81. Spurr NK, Highes D, Goodfellow PN, Brook JD, Padua RA. Chromosomal assignment of c-*mel*, a human transforming oncogene, to chromosome 19 (p13.2-q13.20). Somat Cell Genet 1986; 12:637-640.

82. Albino AP, Sozzi G, Nanus DM, Jhanwar SC, Houghton AN. Malignant transformation of human melanocytes: Induction of a complete melanoma phenotype and genotype. Oncogene 1992; 7:2315-2321.

83. Albino AP, Houghton AN, Eisinger M, Lee JS, Kantor RRS, Oliff AI, Old LJ. Class II major histocompatibility antigen expression in human melanocytes transformed by Harvey murine sarcoma virus (Ha-MSV) and Kirsten MSV (Ki-MSV) retroviruses. J Exp Med 1986; 164:1710.

84. Demetri DG, Ernst TJ, Pratt ES, Zenzie BW, Rheinwald JG, Grifit JD. Expression of RAS oncogene in cultured human cells alters the transcriptional and post transcriptional regulation of cytokine genes. J Clin Invest 1990; 86:1261-1269.

85. Barnekow A, Paul E, Schartl M. Expression of the c-*src* proto-oncogene in human skin tumors. Cancer Res 1987; 47:235-240.

86. O'Connor TJ, Neufeld E, Bechberger J, Fujita DJ. pp60^{c-src} in human melanocytes and melanoma cells exhibits elevated specific activity and reduced tyrosine 530 phosphorylation compared to human fibroblast pp60^{c-src}. Cell Growth Different 1992; 3:435-442.

87. Linnenbach AJ, Huebner K, Reddy EP, Herlyn M, Parmiter AH, Nowell PC, Koprowski H. Structural alteration in the MYB proto-oncogene and deletion within the gene encoding a-type protein kinase C in human melanoma cell lines. Proc Natl Acad Sci USA 1988; 85:74-78.

88. Dasgupta P, Linnenbach AJ, Giaccia AJ, Stamato TD, Reddy EP. Molecular cloning of the breakpoint region on chromosome 6 in cutaneous malignant melanoma: Evidence for deletion in the c-*myb* locus and translocation of a segment of chromosome 12. Oncogene 1989; 4:1201-1205.

89. Meese E, Meltzer PS, Witkowski CM, Trent J. Molecular mapping of the oncogene *myb* and rearrangements in malignant melanoma. Genes, Chromosomes Cancer 1989; 1:88-94.

90. Versteeg R, Noordermeer IA, Krüse-Wolters M, Ruiter DJ, Schrier PI. c-*myc* down-regulates class I HLA expression in human melanomas. EMBO J 1988; 7:1023-1029.

91. Husain Z, Fitzgerald GB, Wick MM. Comparison of cellular proto-oncogene activation and transformation-related activity of human melanocytes and metastatic melanoma. J Invest Dermatol 1990; 95:571-575.

92. Chenevix-Trench G, Martin NG, Ellem KAO. Gene expression in melanoma cell lines and cultured melanocytes: Correlation between levels of c-*src*-1, c-*myc* and p53. 1990; 5:1187-1193.

93. Bauer J, Sokol L, Stribrna J, Kremen M, Krajsova I, Hausner P, Hejnar P. Amplification of N-*myc* oncogene in human melanoma cells. Neoplasma (Czechoslovakia) 1990; 37:233-238.

94. Iwamoto T, Takahashi M, Ito M, Hamatani K, Ohbayashi M, Wajjwalku W, Isobe K-I, Nakashima I. Aberrant melanogenesis and melanocytic tumor development in transgenic mice that carry a metallothionein/*ret* fusion gene. EMBO J 1991; 10:3167-3175.

95. Taniguchi M, Iwamoto T, Nakashima I, Nakayama A, Ohbayashi M, Matsuyama M, Takahashi M. Establishment and characterization of a malignant melanocytic tumor cell line expressing the *ret* oncogene. Oncogene 1992; 7:1491-1496.

96. Yamanishi DT, Buckmeier JA, Meyskens FL Jr. Expression of c-*jun*, *jun*-B, and c-*fos* proto-oncogenes in human primary melanocytes and metastatic melanomas. J Invest Dermatol 1991; 97:349-353.

97. Steeg PS, Bevilacqua G, Kopper L, Thorgeirsson UP, Talmadge JE, Liotta LA, Sobel ME. Evidence for a novel gene associated with low tumor metastatic potential. J Natl Cancer Inst 1988; 80:200-204.

98. Florenes VA, Aamdal S, Myklebost O, Maelandsmo GM, Bruland OS, Fodstad O. Levels of *nm23* messenger RNA in metastatic malignant melanomas: Inverse correlation to disease progression. Cancer Res 1992; 52:6088-6091.

99. Leone A, Flatow U, King CR, Sandeen MA, Margulies IM, Liotta LA, Steeg PS. Reduced tumor incidence, metastatic potential, and cytokine responsiveness of *nm23*-transfected melanoma cells. Cell 1991; 65:25-35.

100. Frisch SM. Antioncogenic effect of adenovirus *E1A* in human tumor cells. Proc Natl Acad Sci USA 1991; 88:9077-81.

101. Anders F. Contributions of the Gordon-Kosswig melanoma system to the present concept of neoplasia. Pigment Cell Research 1991; 3:7-29.

102. Wittbrodt J, Adam D, Malitschek B, Mäueler W, Raulf F, Telling A, Robertson SM, Schartl M. Novel putative receptor tyrosine kinase encoded by the melanoma-inducing *Tu* locus in *Xiphophorus*. Nature 1989; 341:415-421.

103. Adam D, Dimitrijevic N, Schartl M. Tumor suppression in *Xiphophorus* by an accidentally acquired promoter. Science 1993; 259:816-819.

104. Levine AJ, Momand J, Finlay CA. The p53 tumor suppressor gene. Nature 1991; 351:453-456.

105. Hollstein M, Sidransky D, Vogelstein B, Harris CC. p53 mutations in human cancers. Science 1991; 253:49-53.

106. Rodrigues NR, Rosan A, Smith MEF, Kerr IB, Bodmer WF, Gannon JV, Lane DP. p53 mutations in colorectal cancer. Proc Natl Acad Sci USA 1990; 87:7555-7559.

107. Campo E, Calle-Martin O, Miquel R, Palacin A, Romero M, Fabregat V, Vives J, Cardesa A, Yague J. Loss of heterozygosity of p53 gene and p53 protein expression in human colorectal carcinomas. Cancer Res 1991; 51:4436-4442.

108. Thompson AM, Anderson TJ, Condie A, Prosser J, Chetty U, Carter DC, Evans HJ, Steel CM. p53 allele losses, mutations and expression in breast cancer and their relationship to clinicopathological parameters. Int J Cancer 1992; 50:528-532.

109. Coles C, Condie A, Chetty U, Steel CM, Evans HJ, Prosser J. p53 mutations in breast cancer. Cancer Res 1992; 52:5291-5298.

110. Nigro JM, Baker SJ, Preisinger AC, Jessup JM, Hostetter R, Cleary K, Bigner SH, Davidson N, Baylin S, Devilee P, Glover T, Collins FS, Weston A, Modali R, Harris CC, Vogelstein B. Mutations in the p53 gene occur in diverse human tumour types. Nature 1989; 3342:705-708.

111. Mulligan LM, Matlashewski GJ, Scrable HJ, Cavanee WK. Mechanisms of p53 loss in human sarcomas. Proc Natl Acad Sci USA 1990; 87:5863-5867.

112. Malkin D, Li FP, Strong LC, Fraumeni JF Jr, Nelson CE, Kim DH, Kassel J, Gryka MA,

Bischoff FZ, Tainsky MA, Friend SH. Germ line p53 mutations in a familial syndrome of breast cancer, sarcomas, and other neoplasms. Science 1990; 250:1233-1238.

113. Brash DE, Rudolph JA, Simon JA, Lin A, McKenna GJ, Baden HP, Halperin AJ, Ponten J. A role for sunlight in skin cancer: UV induced p53 mutations in squamous cell carcinoma. Proc Natl Acad Sci USA 1991; 88:10124-10128.

114. Brash DE, Ziegler A, Simon JA, Kunala S. A UV mutation spectrum in the p53 gene in basal cell carcinoma of the skin. 83rd annual meeting of the American Association for Cancer Research, San Diego, 1992. In Proceedings Am Assoc Cancer Res 33: 671.

115. Stretch JR, Gatter KC, Ralfkiaer E, Lane DP, Harris AL. Expression of mutant p53 in melanoma. Cancer Res 1991; 51:5976-5979.

116. Volkenandt M, Schlegel U, Nanus DM, Albino AP. Mutational analysis of the human p53 gene in malignant melanoma. Pigment Cell Res 1991; 4:35-40.

117. Weiss J, Schwechheimer K, Cavanee WK, Herlyn M, Arden KC. Mutation and expression of the p53 gene in malignant melanoma cell lines. Int J Cancer, In press.

118. Miller HJ. Mutagenic specificity of ultraviolet light. J Mol Biol 1985; 182:45-68.

119. Besmer P, Murphy PC, George PC, Qui F, Bergold PJ, Lederman L, Snyder HW, Brodeur D, Zuckerman EE, Hardy WD. A new acute transforming feline retrovirus and relationship of its oncogene v-*kit* with the protein kinase gene family. Nature 1986; 320:415-421.

120. Chabot B, Stephenson DA, Chapman VM, Besmer P, Bernstein A. The proto-oncogene c-*kit* encoding a transmembrane tyrosine kinase receptor maps to the mouse *W* locus. Nature 1988; 335:88-89.

121. Geissler EN, Ryan MA, Housman DE. The dominant-white spotting (*W*) locus of the mouse encodes the c-*kit* proto-oncogene. Cell 1988; 55:185-192.

122. Nocka K, Majumder S, Chabot B, Ray P, Cervone M, Bernstein A, Besmer P. Expression of c-*kit* gene products in known cellular targets of *W* mutations in normal and *W* mutant mice — evidence for an impaired c-*kit* kinase in mutant mice. Genes Dev 1989; 3:816-826.

123. Nocka K, Tan JC, Chiu TY, Ray P, Traktman P, Besmer P. Molecular bases of dominant negative and loss of function mutations at the murine c-*kit*/white spotting locus W37, Wv, W41, W. EMBO J 1990; 9:1805-1813.

124. Reith AD, Rottapel R, Giddens E, Brady C, Forrester L, Bernstein A. *W* mutant mice with mild or severe developmental defects contain distinct point mutations in the kinase domain of the c-*kit* transmembrane receptor. Genes Dev 1990; 4:390-400.

125. Tan JC, Nocka K, Ray P, Traktman P, Besmer P. The dominant W42 spotting phenotype results from a missense mutation in the c-*kit* receptor kinase. Science 1990; 247:209-212.

126. Brannan CI, Lyman SD, Williams DE, Eisenman J, Anderson D, Cosman D, Bedell MA, Jenkins NA, Copeland NG. Steel-Dickie mutation encodes a c-*kit* ligand lacking transmembrane and cytoplasmic domains. Proc Natl Acad Sci USA 1991; 88:4671-4674.

127. Flanagan JG, Chan DG, Leder P. Transmembrane form of the *kit* ligand growth factor is determined by alternative splicing and is missing in the Sld mutant. Cell 1991; 64:1025-1035.

128. Nishikawa S, Kusakabe M, Yoshinaga K, Ogawa M, Hayashi S-I, Kunisada T, Era T, Sakakura T, Nishikawa S-I. *In utero* manipulation of coat color formation by a monoclonal anti-c-*kit* antibody: Two distinct waves of c-*kit*-dependency during melanocyte development. EMBO J 1991; 10:2111-2118.

129. Giebel LB, Spritz RA. Mutation of the c-*kit* (mast/stem cell growth factor receptor) proto-oncogene in human piebaldism. Proc Natl Acad Sci USA 1992; 88:8696-8699.

130. Spritz RA, Giebel LB, Holmes SA. Dominant negative and loss of function mutations of the c-*kit* (mast/stem cell growth factor receptor) proto-oncogene in human piebaldism. Am J Hum Genet 1992; 50:261-269.

131. Lassam N, Bickford. Loss of c-*kit* expression in cultured melanoma cells. Oncogene 1992; 7:51-56.

132. Natali PG, Nicotra MR, Winkler AB, Cavaliere R, Bigotti A, Ulrich A. Progression of human cutaneous melanoma is associated with loss of expression of c-*kit* proto-oncogene receptor. Int J Cancer 1992; 52:197-201.

133. Funasaka Y, Boulton T, Cobb M, Yarden Y,

Fan B, Lyman S, Williams DE, Anderson DM, Zakut R, Mishima Y, Halaban R. c-*kit*-kinase induces a cascade of protein tyrosine phosphorylation in normal human melanocytes in response to mast cell growth factor and stimulates mitogen-activated protein kinase but is down-regulated in melanomas. Mol Biol Cell 1992; 3:197-209.

134. Larue L, Dougherty N, Porter S, Mintz B. Spontaneous malignant transformation of melanocytes explanted from Wf/Wf mice with a *Kit* kinase-domain mutation. Proc Natl Acad Sci USA 1992; 89:7816-7820.

135. Morrison-Graham K, West-Johnsrud L, Weston JA. Extracellular matrix from normal but not *steel* mutant mice enhances melanogenesis in cultured mouse neural crest cells. Dev Biol 1990; 139:299-307.

136. Lehmann JM, Riethmüller G, Johnson JP. *Nck*, a melanoma cDNA encoding a cytoplasmic protein consisting of the *src* homology units SH2 and SH3. Nucleic Acids Res 1990; 18:1048.

137. Chou MM, Fajardo JE, Hanafusa H. The SH2- and SH3-containing *nck* protein transforms mammalian fibroblasts in the absence of elevated phosphotyrosine levels. Mol Cell Biol 1992; 12:5834-5842.

138. Li W, Hu P, Skolnik Y, Ullrich A, Schlessinger J. The SH2 and SH3 domain-containing *nck* protein is oncogenic and a common target for phosphorylation by different surface receptors. Mol Cell Biol 1992; 12:5824-5833.

139. Park D, Rhee SG. Phosphorylation of *nck* in response to a variety of receptors, phorbol myristate acetate, and cyclic AMP. Mol Cell Biol 1992; 12:5816-5823.

140. The I, Murthy AE, Hannigan GE, Jacoby LB, Menon AG, Gusella JF, Bernards A. Neurofibromatosis type 1 gene mutations in neuroblastoma. Nature 1993; 3:62-66.

141. Andersen LB, Fountain JW, Gutmann DH, Tarlé SA, Glover TW, Dracopoli NC, Housman DE, Collins FS. Mutations in the neurofibromatosis 1 gene in sporadic malignant melanoma cell lines. Nature Genetics 1993; 3:118-121.

142. Seizinger BR. *NF1*: A prevalent cause of tumorigenesis in human cancer? Nature Genetics 1993; 3:97-99.

143. Hutchins JT, Deans RJ, Mitchell MS, Uchiyama C, Kan-Mitchell J. Novel gene sequences expressed by human melanoma cells identified by molecular subtraction. Cancer Res 1991; 51:1418-1425.

144. Weterman MA, Stoopen GM, van Muijen GN, Kuznicki J, Ruiter DJ, Bloemers HP. Expression of calcyclin in human melanoma cell lines correlates with metastatic behavior in nude mice. Cancer Res 1992; 52:1291-1296.

CHAPTER 4

Tumor Progression in the Melanocytic System

PRECURSOR STAGES OF MELANOCYTES

Melanocytes are pigmented cells located in the basal layer of the epidermis, the infundibulum and the bulb of hair sheaths, the choroid of the eye, certain mucous membranes, and the leptomeninges. These neuroectoderm-derived cells leave the neural crest 2-3 weeks after fertilization and migrate through the embryonal dermis to reach the epidermis by 8-10 weeks. These immature precursor cells, melanoblasts, do not actively produce pigment until after birth, except in some areas of the nipples and the genitalia. Ultrastructurally, these cells possess premelanosomes (grade I and II melanosomes; melanosome precursors lacking melanin) but do not exhibit tyrosinase activity.[1] The pathway of maturation of melanocytes, as summarized in Table 2, is unclear. Experimental evidence to delineate each maturation stage is incomplete, but it appears that melanoblasts undergo at least two precursor stages before maturing. Intermediate cell types, *premelanocytes*, can be isolated, cultured, and cloned from neonatal human skin.[2] These cells are unpigmented or slightly pigmented, and contain grade I and II melanosomes (premelanosomes). The vast majority of these cells are tyrosinase-negative; however, tyrosinase and pigmentation can be activated by elevating the pH of culture medium from 6.8 to 7.4 and supplementing the medium with 1 mM tyrosine, the precursor of melanin. Following these manipulations, pigmentation of these unpigmented or barely pigmented clones occurs gradually.[2] The progressive stabilization of melanin synthesis has led to the concept of gradual commitment of these cells in their maturation pathway.[3,4] Bennett[3] hypothesized that stable commitment occurs when melanocytes become pigmented.

In the mouse embryo, melanocyte precursor migration to the skin has been increasingly studied in *W (c-kit)* mutant mice (see Chapter 3). Blocking of the biological activity of c-*kit* through gene mutations or with specific antibodies has proven that c-*kit* plays a determining role in the melanocyte migration process.

The putative equivalents of the premelanocyte in vivo can be found in the outer sheath of the hair follicles, which contains amelanotic melanocytes. By contrast, pigmented melanocytes are characteristically located in the wall of the hair follicle pilary canal (infundibulum) and in the pigmented portion of the hair bulb. It is possible that the amelanotic melanocyte cells, under the stimulus of epidermal regeneration and/or UV irradiation, undergo serial divisions, migrate and mature into dendritic, pigmented melanocytes.

Mature melanocytes are multidendritic pigmented cells located mainly in the basal layer of the epidermis. Within the epidermis, melanocytes have a symbiotic relationship with associated keratinocytes and form the epidermal melanin unit.[6] Mature melanocytes are tyrosinase-positive and produce pigment through the action of this enzyme. These cells contain melanosomes of all stages of maturation and transport pigment to adjacent keratinocytes.

Table 2. Maturation of melanocytes

Cell stage	Phenotype	Location
Melanoblast ↓↑ ↓↑	?	Migration from neural crest
Early premelanocyte ↓↑ ↓↑	Round, noncharacteristic; noncharacteristic; tyrosinase⁻ (a); pigmentation⁻; proliferating (b).	Fetal dermis; outer sheath of hair follicle: adult dermis (?)
Intermediate ??	Uni- or bipolar; premelanosomes; tyrosinase activity⁻(a); pigmentation (±); proliferating (b).	Fetal dermis; adult dermis (?): infundibulum of hair follicle
Melanocyte	Bi- to tripolar, or multidendritic; premelanosomes and melanosomes; tyrosinase activity⁺; pigmentation⁺; proliferating (b).	Basal layers of skin; infundibulum and bulb of hair follicle; (eye mucous membranes, leptomeninges)

from Valyi-Nagy and Herlyn (1991).
Tyrosinase activity (a) and proliferation (b) can be specifically modulated by culture conditions and forced regeneration.

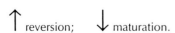 ↑ reversion;   ↓ maturation.

CLINICAL AND PATHOLOGICAL EVIDENCE FOR TUMOR PROGRESSION

The clinical and histopathological features of tumor progression in the human melanocytic system have been described in detail.[7-12] As illustrated in Figure 4, melanoma can develop from precursor or mature melanocytes and progress through different stages starting with benign nevi, which are congenital or acquired, to dysplastic lesions. Potentially, nevi are capable of evolving into malignant melanomas, an evolution that has been observed in 1.1% of small congenital nevi and 6.3% of giant congenital nevi.[7] The proportion of melanoma cases associated with a small congenital nevus might be as high as 14.9%.[13] Among acquired nevi, cells of the familial dysplastic nevus syndrome appear to have a high probability for malignant transformation,[7,8] and it is estimated that more than 85% of familial melanomas arise from precursor lesions.[14]

Melanocytic nevi can be regarded as benign neoplasms of melanocytes.[12] They are almost ubiquitous in humans, appearing first in early childhood, reaching a maximum count in young adults and declining in older age groups. Histopathological observations suggest that nevi can regress due to an active immune response [15] or through a differentiation pathway leading to senescence and atrophy.[16,17] This regression of common acquired nevi through a differentiation pathway is a frequent phenomenon. Sagebiel [18] and Elder et al[12] have estimated that each of the 160 million adult Caucasians in the United States have approximately 20 nevi, resulting in a "nevus population" of 3.2 billion (Fig. 5). Progression among nevi from ordinary to dysplastic nevi is uncommon. Progression beyond benign lesions is even more rare, since only 30,000 melanomas develop per annum (about 1 per 110,000 original nevi).

The term "dysplastic nevus" representing the intermediate lesions of Figure 4 has recently been redefined by a consensus conference,[19] and is now described as "atypical mole" and "nevus with architectural disorder," terms originally used by Clark[7] and Greene.[8] Elder et al[12] have now suggested the terms "melanocytic (histologic) dysplasia" and "clinically atypical (melanocytic) nevi," i.e., the discussion on nevus definitions is ongoing.

The clinical features of nevi are described in terms of size, profile, border and color.[20-23] Dysplastic nevi are usually at least 5 mm in diameter, with a macular component, an unclear border and an irregular color. Histologically, the lesions contain randomly atypical melanocytes with large nuclei, and architectural changes are due to irregular connective tissue arrangement. Dysplastic nevus lesions are often surrounded in the dermis by lymphocytes.[11]

Clark[11] has distinguished between in situ melanomas, which have large epitheloid cells with large and hyperchromatic nuclei, and radial growth phase (RGP) melanomas, which have the same features as in situ melanomas except that individual melanocytic cells have invaded the dermis. RGP melanomas are often larger than 10 mm in diameter, and highly asymmetrical with a pagetoid spread expanding into the stratum corneum. Mitotic cells can be seen in the epidermis but not in the dermis. The lymphocytic infiltrate is band-like in the dermis. In situ/RGP melanoma has also been termed lentigo maligna, atypical melanocytic proliferation, and pagetoid melanocytic proliferation.[19] All of these early melanomas can be effectively treated by conservative surgery. Of 147 cases studied over >10 years, none recurred or metastasizied.[11] The lack of metastasis formation of RGP melanomas cannot be predicted from histological features of the lesions since infiltrating cells are found in the dermis which suggests that these melanomas have invasive capability but they do not survive even if they successfully enter the vasculature.

Invasive primary melanomas are currently divided into four subtypes:[19] 1) superficial spreading melanoma, which is the most common subtype and can be located on any anatomic site; 2) nodular melanoma, which presents as elevated or polyploid lesion, and is uniform in pigmentation and frequently ulcerated; 3) lentigo maligna melanoma, a macular lesion on sun-exposed skin (head, neck), often found in patients with in situ/RGP

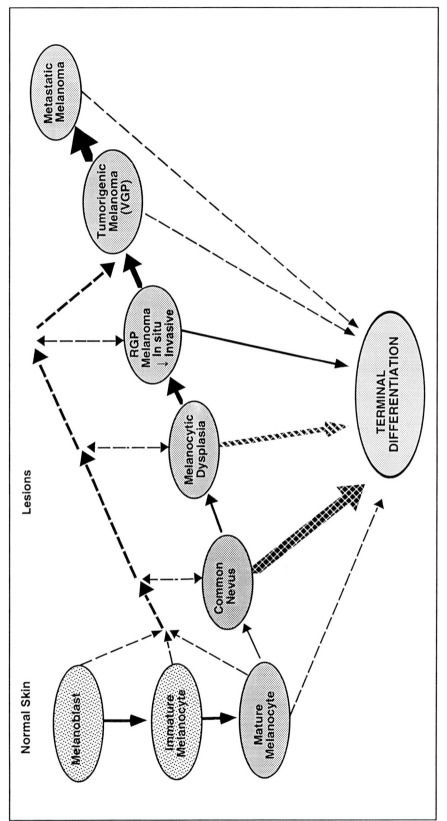

Fig. 4. Stepwise tumor progression based on models by Clark[11] and Elder.[12] Precursor cells of melanocytes mature functionally into cells that can transport pigment through dendritic processes to keratinocytes. Generally, mature melanocytes in situ show no detectable proliferation. In vitro, melanocytes proliferate and may differentiate into a fibroblast-like cell type. Progression of normal cells to melanoma cells may occur at any maturation stage or tumor progression may be sequential, nevus to dysplasia to melanoma. Lesions composed of cells undergoing differentiation regress until they disappear. Nevus cells may persist in situ or spontaneously differentiate along pathways which have been defined histopathologically as Schwannian differentiation and experimentally as fibroblast-like differentiation. Differentiation of melanoma cells is rare but may occur along the same pathways.

melanoma; and 4) acral lentiginous melanoma, which is presented as a darkly pigmented, flat to nodular lesion on palms, soles, and subungually.

The clinical and pathological features of superficial spreading melanoma have been described by Clark and co-workers[10] as vertical growth phase (VGP) melanomas which, unlike RGP melanomas, are able to metastasize. VGP lesions enlarge along the radii of an imperfect circle and expand into the dermis. Patients with VGP melanomas have an 8-year survival rate of 71%. A number of parameters can be applied to predict with 90% accuracy survival of patients with VGP primary melanoma over an 8-year period.[10] Survival prediction can be enhanced by applying a multivariable logistic regression model, including the following parameters: 1) mitotic rate, 2) tumor thickness, and 3) presence or absence of infiltrating lymphocytes (the

three most important predictors), 4) anatomic site (trunk or extremities), 5) sex (female or male) and 6) regression (presence or absence), see Table 3.

Additional parameters which significantly predict lower survival are microscopic satellites (absence vs presence), ulceration (absence vs presence), vascular invasion (absence vs presence), plasma cells (absence vs presence), and nodular growth (absence vs presence). These latter parameters were not included in the mathematical model of survival prediction.[10] This model provides not only valuable information for the clinical follow-up of patients, but also helps to direct research regarding the critical components of tumor progression.

Metastasis is the final step of tumor progression. In the study by Clark,[11] 18% of metastases disseminated only to the regional lymph node, 39% of analyzed cases showed dissemination initial to the regional lymph

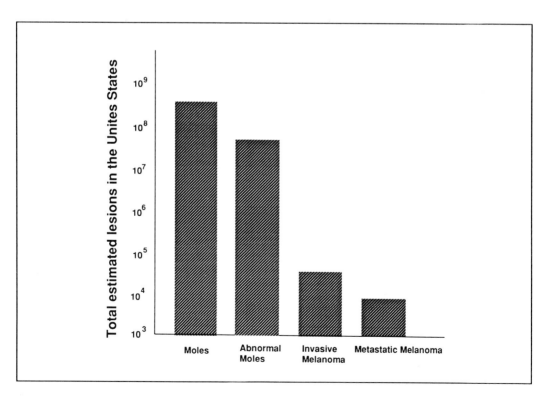

Fig. 5. Estimates on the natural history of melanocytic lesions assuming a total population of 160,000,000 adult Caucasians in the United States with an average of 20 nevi per individual. The number of abnormal nevi is 10-fold less, and that of invasive melanoma 100,000-fold less (1 per 110,000 original nevi).

nodes followed by blood hematogenous metastases, and 43% of the cases showed blood vascular metastasis without apparent involvement of the lymphatic system. Lung, brain, and liver are the preferred sites, but metastatic melanomas can be found in virtually any anatomic site.

IN VITRO STUDIES WITH MELANOCYTES FROM DIFFERENT STAGES OF TUMOR PROGRESSION

NORMAL MELANOCYTES

The development of isolation methods and special culture media for selective growth and long-term maintenance of melanocytes has been a major basic contribution to an understanding of pigment cell biology.[24] For

almost 30 years isolation and in vitro growth of human melanocytes had been attempted,[25-28] but it was only in 1982 that pure cultures of normal human melanocytes were reproducibly established to yield large quantities of cells for biological, biochemical, and molecular analysis. Eisinger and Marko[29] found that the tumor promoter phorbol 12-myristate-13-acetate (PMA) and the intracellular cyclic adenosine 3',5' monophosphate (cAMP) enhancer cholera toxin were strong mitogens for melanocytes. The first report of a physiologic melanocyte mitogen was provided by Gilchrest et al,[30] who used bovine hypothalamus extracts and cholera toxin for melanocyte culture. The recent, rapid development of tissue culture methods has led to effective, standardized procedures for the culture of human epidermal melanocytes. Information obtained from normal melanocytes

Table 3. Tumor and host factors associated with survival of melanoma patients with clinical stage I vertical growth phase (VGP) primary melanoma.

Parameter	Category	(Adjusted odds ratios for survival)
Thickness	< 1.70 (mm)	4.04
	> 1.70	1.00
Mitotic rate	0.0 (per mm)	11.69
	0.1-6.0	3.49
	> 6.0	1.00
Site	Extremities	3.80
	Head, neck, trunk, subungual	1.00
Tumor infiltrating lymphocytes (TIL)	Brisk	11.31
	Nonbrisk	3.51
	Absent	1.00
Sex	Female	2.92
	Male	1.00
Regression	Absent or incomplete	2.79
	Present	1.00

Modified from Clark et al, 1989.

Table 4. Factors that modulate melanocyte growth and/or morphology in culture[a]

Name	Main type of action
Growth factors	
bFGF	Growth stimulation
K-FGF/Hst-1	Growth stimulation
FGF-5	Growth stimulation
FGF-6 C	Growth stimulation
MGF/SCF	Growth stimulation
HGF/SF	Growth stimulation, motility
Insulin/IGF-1	Growth stimulation
EGF/TGF-α	Growth stimulation,[b] motility
TGF-β	Growth inhibition
Calcium and cation binding proteins	
Ca^2+ (1.0-2.0 mM)	Growth stimulation
Ceruloplasmin (Cu^2+)	Growth stimulation
Transferrin (Fe^2+)	Growth stimulation
Enhancers of cAMP	
α-MSH	Growth stimulation, pigmentation
FSH	Growth stimulation, pigmentation
Cholera toxin	Growth stimulation, pigmentation
Forskolin	Growth stimulation, pigmentation
Isobutyl methylxanthine (IBMX)	Growth stimulation, pigmentation
Activators of protein kinase C	
TPA	Growth stimulation
PDBu	Growth stimulation
Inflammatory mediators and cytokines	
Leukotriene LTC4	Growth stimulation, motility
Endothelin-1	Growth stimulation, motility
IL-1	Growth inhibition, pigmentation, matrix protein
IL-6	Growth inhibition, pigmentation, matrix protein
TNF-α	Growth inhibition, pigmentation, matrix protein?
Prostaglandins E2, D2, F_{2a}	Pigmentation, growth stimulation
Histamine	Morphology
Miscellaneous compounds	
Dibutyrl cAMP	Growth promotion/morphology
1,25(OH)2 vitamin-D_3/25(OH) vitamin-D3	Morphology/growth promotion?
Extracellular matrix (ECM)	Morphology/growth modulation?
Physical agents	
Ultraviolet light (UV-B), UV-C)	Growth promotion/morphology

[a] Modified from Valyi-Nagy and Herlyn, 1991.
[b] Only during the initial passages of melanocytes.

has provided evidence of constitutive activation of signaling pathways in melanoma cells.

A number of studies have led to the delineation of four groups of chemically defined melanocyte mitogens: 1) peptide growth factors, 2) calcium and cation binding proteins, 3) enhancers of intracellular levels of cAMP, and 4) activators of protein kinase C. Ultraviolet light (UV-B) appears to be the only physical mitogen with a known growth stimulatory effect.[31-34] Table 4 summarizes the factors that modulate the growth of melanocytes in culture.

PEPTIDE GROWTH FACTORS

The main growth-promoting polypeptide in bovine brain (hypothalamus) and pituitary extracts is basic fibroblast growth factor (bFGF).[35,36] Basic FGF can exert its stimulatory effect only in combination with either cAMP-enhancing components or activators of protein kinase C. Besides bFGF, a number of other members of the FGF family are mitogenic for melanocytes. These include KGF and FGF-6.[37] Additionally mast cell growth factor (MGF), also termed stem cell growth factor (SCF) or steel[38] and hepatocyte growth factor (HGF) or scatter factor (SF) have growth stimulatory activity and induce motility of melanocytes.[39,40] Insulin-like growth factor-I (IGF-I) and insulin share a similar growth-promoting effect, since they bind to the same cell surface (IGF-I) receptor. However, it has been shown that the affinity of IGF-I for this receptor on melanoma cells is approximately 100-fold higher.[41] EGF supports the growth of melanocytes during the initial passage, but is not mitogenic for established cultures.[42,43] Transforming growth factor-alpha (TGF-α) has a similar, if not identical, effect, whereas TGF-β inhibits melanocyte growth.[44]

CALCIUM AND CATION BINDING PROTEINS

Ca^{2+} is an important cation in melanocyte growth media. Its optimal concentration is 1.0-2.0 mM. Reduction of calcium concentration in medium to 0.03 mM reduces cell growth by approximately 50%.[45] Cation binding proteins such as tyrosinase (copper), ceruloplasmin (copper), or transferrin (iron) are mitogenic for melanocytes.[45]

COMPOUNDS THAT ENHANCE INTRACELLULAR LEVELS OF cAMP

A great variety of compounds of diverse origin have been described to be mitogens for melanocytes in cultures.[45] Alpha-melanocyte stimulating hormone (α-MSH) is a very strong mitogen in chemically defined melanocyte growth medium for human melanocytes, but the mechanisms of action are not clear. Conversely, β-MSH probably has no effect on human melanocytes.[46] Forskolin and follicle-stimulating hormone, after increasing the intracellular level of cAMP, also increase the binding of insulin to the cells.[47]

PROTEIN KINASE C ACTIVATORS

Protein kinase C-activating phorbol esters are very strong mitogens for melanocytes. 12-0-Tetradecanoyl-phorbol-13-acetate (TPA) is lipophilic, so it cannot be easily removed from cells by washing. 20-Oxo-phorbol-12-13-dibutyrate (PDBu) is a similar, but more hydrophilic, derivative. Besides their mitogenic effect, phorbol esters also drastically alter the morphology of melanocytes. Withdrawal of phorbol ester from melanocyte growth medium induces a 'fibroblastoid' morphology and greatly decreases growth rate. This change is reversible if the growth medium is replenished with phorbol ester within 14 days. Thus, these compounds are necessary for maintaining not only cell proliferation, but also the characteristic bi- or tripolar phenotype (Fig. 6A).[29]

INFLAMMATORY MEDIATORS AND CYTOKINES

Inflammatory mediators and cytokines often modulate not only melanocyte proliferation, but also production of pigment.[48-53] These compounds can also regulate migration of cells. Leukotrienes, endothelins and prostaglandins are growth stimulators, whereas IL-1 and IL-6 and TNF-α are growth inhibitors. Only the leukotrienes LTD_4 and LTC_4 are effective melanocyte mitogens without the addition of other mitogens.[49] They appear to involve protein kinase A activation, because they are inhibited by a protein kinase

A inhibitor.[50] It has been hypothesized that inflammatory mediators such as leukotriene C_4 contribute to nevus development because they induce loss of contact inhibition and formation of structures resembling tumor spheroids.[49] Endothelins trigger an increase in intracellular calcium levels and inositol-1,4,5-triphosphate and may stimulate melanocytes through this second messenger pathway.[51,52] Prostaglandins can act as modulators and/or mediators in pigmented cells. Prostaglandin F_{2a} was shown to have a strong stimulatory effect on melanocytes, using chemically defined media.[45] Treating cells with prostaglandin E_2 results in only morphological changes.[53]

MISCELLANEOUS COMPOUNDS THAT AFFECT MELANOCYTE GROWTH AND/OR MORPHOLOGY

Dibutyryl cAMP (dbcAMP) is a very strong inducer of dendrite formation (Fig. 6B and C). The number of dendritic processes increased about 10-fold within 4-6 days of dbcAMP treatment.[45] This morphologic effect is reversible; melanocytes reassume their bi- or tripolar morphology 4-8 days after the removal of dbcAMP from medium. dbcAMP also has a growth-promoting effect when used together with cholera toxin.[54]

Histamine, produced in the skin by mast cells, is also stimulatory for cultured melanocytes.[55] In a dose-dependent fashion, histamine increases both the amount of tyrosinase and the size of melanocytes, and cells become more dendritic. These changes can already be observed 6 hours after supplementing the medium with histamine.

1,25-dihydroxyvitamin D_3 (1,25(OH)$_2$D$_3$) and 25-hydroxyvitamin D_3 (25(OH)D$_3$) are the active derivatives of vitamin D_3. The precursor of this hormone is synthesized in the basal layer of the skin upon exposure to UV light. Normal human melanocytes, melanoma cells, and keratinocytes have the biochemical capacity to convert vitamin D_3 into its active hydroxylated metabolites.[56-58] Topical treatment of mice with cholecalciferol or 1,25(OH)$_2$D$_3$ increases the number of pigmented cells. This phenomenon is due either to the reactivation of residing melanocytes or to a direct mitogenic effect. The

effect of the topical treatment was blocked by simultaneous oral treatment of the mice with indomethacin. In cultured human melanocytes, 1,25(OH)$_2$D$_3$ and to a lesser extent 25(OH)D$_3$, cause a marked decrease in tyrosinase activity.

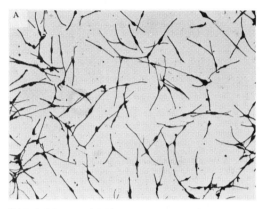

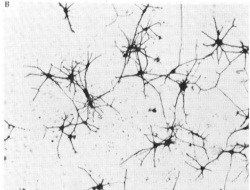

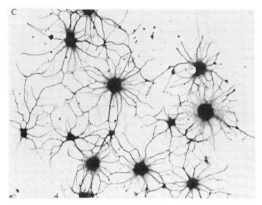

Fig. 6. Normal melanocytes in culture. A, melanocytes in the presence of complete medium (W489 medium supplemented with TPA, FCS, insulin, and EGF). B and C, melanocytes in complete medium supplemented with dibutyryl cAMP which leads to extensive arborization as in skin.

The differences between the results obtained from animal experiments and in vitro studies might rest in the lack in cultures of keratinocytes and Langerhans cells, which may be the source of other undefined mediators. It has also been shown that human melanocytes in culture express receptors to vitamin D_3. The isolated receptor molecule was found to migrate in the 53-kDa region.[59] The vitamin D_3 receptor appears in the nucleus linked to the retinoid acid receptor.

Human epidermal melanocytes cultured on extracellular matrix (ECM)-coated plastic surfaces develop flatter and larger cell bodies, and melanin production is enhanced. Pigmented human melanoma cells are not affected by the presence of ECM.[60]

Melanocytes from newborn foreskin grown in the presence of insulin, EGF, pituitary extract, fetal calf serum, and TPA have doubling times of 2-4 days for 40-60 doublings. Heavily pigmented cells may senesce after 20-30 doublings. Dendricity increases at higher passage levels. Normal melanocytes have a diploid karyotype and are non-tumorigenic in athymic nude mice. These cells do not proliferate anchorage independently in soft agar.[42] The minimal additives to W489 medium for normal melanocyte proliferation are insulin, TPA, α-MSH or other cAMP enhancers, and bFGF (Table 5). If cells are cultured on gelatin as a substrate for better attachment, they can be maintained for several months. Other investigators have developed similar media except that the cAMP enhancer may vary.[37]

Growth, morphology and antigenic phenotype of melanocytes is regulated by undifferentiated keratinocytes through cell-cell contact.[43] In co-cultures allowing physical contact between undifferentiated keratinocytes and melanocytes, melanocytes are positioned singly among keratinocytes, become multidendritic, and establish contact with surrounding epithelial cells. Both cell types proliferate and the cell ratios remain constant over a 14-day period. By contrast, melanocyte proliferation is not supported by conditioned medium of differentiated keratinocyte cultures.

The mechanism of regulation of growth and antigen expression by cell contact remains unclear. Cell surface protein or carbo-hydrate structures, as well as direct exchange of cytoplasmic material, may play a role in the regulation of melanocytic proliferation and antigen expression by keratinocytes. The expression of melanoma-associated antigens on cultured melanocytes in the absence of keratinocytes may result from the loss of direct contact with undifferentiated, basal-type keratinocytes because conditioned medium alone or undifferentiated keratinocytes cannot modulate antigen expression on melanocytes.[61] Since transformed melanocytes migrate from the basal layer of the epidermis to the dermis, it is conceivable that the separation of melanocytes and keratinocytes disrupts the communication between these two cell types and may represent an early step in the pathogenesis of melanoma, allowing proliferation of melanocytes and the expression of new surface structures. It is likely that melanoma-associated antigens such as 9-O-acetyl-GD_3, a 120-kDa protein, and melanotransferrin are expressed on melanocytes as a function of increased proliferation and migration away from keratinocytes rather than transformation.

NEVUS CELLS

Cells from congenital and common acquired nevi can be cultured at a high success rate.[62-68] Nevus cells can be isolated from separate parts of the same lesion: the epidermal, junctional and dermal components.[68] The morphology of nevus cells is similar to that of melanocytes but more heterogeneous because it reflects the histological type and tissue compartment of the nevus from which it is derived.[68] In general, congenital compound nevi yield nevus cells from all the components, with best results obtained with dermal isolates. Lentigo and junctional nevi give poorly growing epidermal and/or junctional cell cultures. Dermal nevus cells live longer than epidermal nevus cells and, at least for congenital compound nevi, the life span of cells in culture seems to be inversely correlated with the age of the donor.

The growth requirements of nevus cells in vitro are similar to those of normal melanocytes. In the presence of serum, even at low concentrations, they do not require pituitary extract. Phorbol ester, although not necessary, maintains a differentiated phenotype in these cells and high growth rate for the life span in culture. Like normal melanocytes, nevus cells are stimulated by TPA (Fig. 7). In the absence of TPA, they lose their pigmentation markers and growth rate slows. However, due to the heterogeneity of nevus cell lines, these changes may occur in a few weeks or over a period of several months. One congenital nevus kept continuously in culture for two years without TPA still exhibits an unaltered proliferative rate and expression of pigmentation markers.[67] If cultured under serum-free conditions, nevus cells, like normal melanocytes, require insulin or IGF-I for growth (Table 5). In contrast to normal melanocytes, nevus cells are less dependent on bFGF.[68] Nevus extracts contain bFGF-like activity and they express bFGF mRNA which is also synthesized by melanoma cells, suggesting that bFGF is synthesized for autocrine growth stimulation.

Like normal melanocytes, nevus cells grown in serum-free medium are stimulated by α-MSH. Unlike for melanocytes, α-MSH cannot be substituted with other compounds that enhance cAMP levels.[68] The mitogenic activity of α-MSH on nevus cells can only be seen in chemically defined medium; in serum-containing medium, α-MSH had no effect.[54]

Nevus cells can grow in soft agar with a colony-forming efficiency varying between 0.1 and 3.7%, but tumor development has not been observed after injection of nevus cells into nude mice previously cultured either in the presence or absence of TPA. Nevus cells maintained in culture for six months to two years have never shown indications of spontaneous malignant transformation.

Common acquired and congenital nevi studied in our laboratory have not shown any karyotypically abnormal clones, whereas cells of two out of eight dysplastic nevi had random clonal karyotypic abnormalities.[69,70] However, the presence of abnormal clones in three out of eight compound nevi examined has been reported.[66]

Table 5. Minimal requirements for growth factors and other mitogens by cultured melanocytic cells[a,b]

Melanocytes	Nevus cells	Primary melanoma cells (VPG)	Metastatic melanoma cells
Insulin (or IGF-I)	Insulin (or IGF-I)	Insulin (or IGF-I)[c]	—
TPA	(TPA)[d]	—[e]	—[e]
α-MSH or other cAMP enhancer	α-MSH	—	—
bFGF[f]	(bFGF)[g]	—	—

[a] FCS is mitogenic for cells from all stages of tumor progression.

[b] EGF is mitogenic for cells from all stages of tumor progression during the first 2-3 weeks only.

[c] Insulin and IGF-I both bind to the IGF-I receptor.

[d] Cells survive longer than melanocytes in absence of TPA.

[e] TPA is inhibitory for primary and metastatic melanoma cells.

[f] Bovine pituitary-derived bFGF is more mitogenic than recombinant bFGF.

[g] Heterogeneous response among cultures, with some cultures independent.

Nevus cells appear to be one step closer than normal melanocytes to developing the growth autonomy that characterizes malignant cells. On the one hand, the differences between nevus and primary melanoma cells in requirements for α-MSH demonstrate the non-malignant nature of nevus cells. On the other hand, the synthesis of bFGF by nevus cells but not normal melanocytes demonstrates their differences from melanocytes and indicates the premalignant nature of nevus cells. These data can be interpreted to support the hypothesis that nevi represent an intermediate stage of tumor progression toward melanoma. The observed differences between nevus cells and newborn foreskin melanocytes are probably not related to body sites, because the biological characteristics of cultured adult melanocytes from different parts of the body are similar to those of newborn foreskin melanocytes, except that adult cells have a shorter life span.

DYSPLASTIC NEVUS CELLS AND RGP PRIMARY MELANOMA CELLS

Little information is available on cultured dysplastic nevus cells. The need for diagnostic material from biopsies leaves only very small specimens for experimental studies and the success rate in cultivation is very low. Moreover, dysplastic nevus and RGP melanoma cultures are phenotypically heterogeneous. Dysplastic nevus cultures may represent only a fraction of the total cultured nevus cells from a given lesion and may be overgrown by common nevus cells. Consequently, cultures may resemble either common acquired nevi or early primary melanomas (Table 6).

In addition to technical problems resulting from the small specimen size available for tissue culture, the majority of RGPs display properties that are not characteristic of other melanocytic cells. The initially dendritic, strongly pigmented but slow-growing

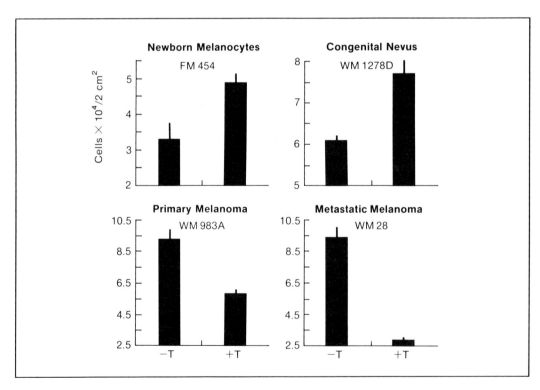

*Fig. 7. Growth of newborn melanocytes and congenital nevus cells (upper panels), and primary and metastatic melanoma cells (lower panels). All cells were cultured in the presence (+T) or absence (-T) of TPA in W489 medium supplemented with insulin, epidermal growth factor, and 2% FCS. 2-3 x 104 cells/cm²
were seeded and the number of cells was determined after 8 days of incubation.*

melanocytic cells are overgrown by a population of flatter, rapidly growing cells which have lost their pigmentation markers, but maintain the expression of some melanoma-associated antigens (see below).[68] These cells show a decreased requirement for medium supplementation, have an extended life span, and grow in soft agar with relatively high colony-forming efficiency. Whether this growing population is truly representative of an early melanoma or is a clone of VGP-type cells already present and selected in culture, has yet to be determined. We have also developed one cell line (WM1650) from a complex primary melanoma lesion that has characteristics of a very early (RGP) primary melanoma. The cells are stimulated by TPA and do not grow anchorage independently in soft agar. However, they have an aneuploid karyotype. When injected into nude mice, cells do not proliferate for several weeks to months, but do remain alive and after 10 months, a 2 x 4 mm

nodule can be isolated that is heavily infiltrated with mouse stromal cells.

VERTICAL GROWTH PHASE PRIMARY AND METASTATIC MELANOMA CELLS

We have established cell lines of more than 30 VGP primary melanomas and more than 250 metastatic melanomas. Examples of cell lines representing early (from patients who have not recurred), intermediate (recurrence after 9 to 84 months), and late primary melanomas (metastases removed at the time of primary melanoma surgery) are given in Table 7. Of cell lines from intermediate and advanced primary melanomas, metastatic cell lines are available from the same patients. The doubling times are shorter for metastatic cells when compared to primary melanoma (Table 8). Metastatic cells have higher colony-forming efficiencies than primary cells when grown either at clonal cell densities or in soft

Table 6. Morphology and growth of nevus and melanoma cells

Common acquired and congenital nevus cells	Dysplastic nevus and RGP melanoma cells	VGP primary melanoma cells	Metastatic melanoma cells
• Bipolar	• Bipolar	• Spindle or cuboidal, similar to metastases	• Spindle or cuboidal
• Pigmented	• Morphological heterogeneity with individual cells having a "transformed" phenotype	• Pigmented in 20-30% of cases	• Morphologic heterogeneity between cultures but not within cultures
• Morphologic heterogeneity		• Morphologic heterogeneity between cultures but not within cultures	
• Induction of dendrites by dibutyryl cAMP less dramatic than in melanocytes and not consistent	• Spontaneous differentiation frequently into nonpigmented, flat cells with no tyrosinase activity		• High cell density/cm²
		• Spontaneous differentiation (20-40% mostly from early lesions)	• Success rate for establishing permanent cell lines: 50-70% (15 h to 5 days doubling time)
• 20-50 doublings (20 h to 14 days doubling time depending on age of donor)	• Possible spontaneous transofrmation in culture		• Rarely spontaneous differentiation (<15%)
	• Poor growth, prolonged survival but no infinite growth	• Success rate for establishing permanent cell lines: 20% (early), 30-40% (intermediate), and 70% (late); 15 h to 7 days doubling times	

agar.[63,71,72] All cell lines of VGP primary melanomas and metastatic melanomas are tumorigenic after injection of $2\text{-}10 \times 10^6$ cells per mouse. The growth rates, however, differ widely (Table 8). Primary melanomas of late lesions have the same growth characteristics as their metastatic counterparts. Cells of primary and metastatic melanomas are maximally stimulated by FCS (Table 9). Metastatic cells can also grow in medium without exogenous growth factors[73] (Fig. 8). Of primary melanoma cells, this can only be achieved with those from advanced lesions (Fig. 8, III). Metastatic cells are stimulated by insulin, EGF, and transferrin which also act synergistically (Table 9). TPA is a growth inhibitor for VGP primary and metastatic cells.

EXPERIMENTAL TUMOR DEVELOPMENT AND PROGRESSION

Normal melanocytes and common acquired nevus cells can be transformed with SV40 T antigen, using either a hybrid virus between SV40 and adenovirus 12 (Ad 12/SV40) or the SV40 T antigen cDNA.[74,75] As shown in Table 10, SV40-transformed melanocytes and nevus cells have several characteristics of spontaneously transformed melanocytes, including growth in soft agar, independence from exogenous growth factors, inhibition by TPA, and an infinite life span (more than 100 doublings). However, the cells are not tumorigenic in nude mice, in contrast to spontaneously transformed VGP

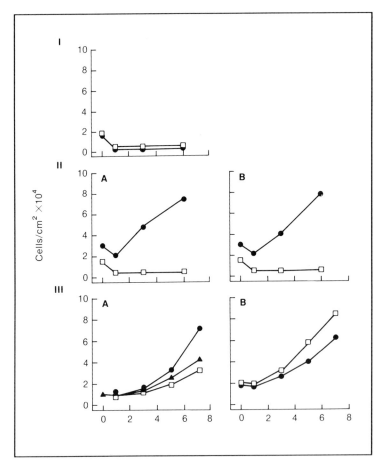

Fig. 8. Growth of primary melanoma cell lines representing early group I, intermediate group II, and advanced group III lesions in serum and growth factor-free W489 medium protein-free medium. Prior to assay, cells were maintained for 4 weeks in protein-free medium to remove residual serum components. Cell number was adjusted to $1\text{-}3 \times 10^4/cm^2$ on day 0 and cells were counted on days 1, 3, 5, and 7. Results are shown for cells lines: WM 793 (□) and WM902B (●) of group I; primary WM115 (□) of group II with autologous metastasis; WM239A (●) (panel A); and primary WM75 (□) with autologous metastasis WM 373 (●) (panel B); primary WM 983A (□) of group III with autologous metastases WM 983B (●) and WM983C (▲) (panel A), and primary WM 1361A (□) with autologous metastasis WM1361C (●) (panel B). [From Kath et al, 1991].

Table 7. Primary and metastatic melanoma cell lines isolated from lesions of patients with long-term clinical follow-up[a]

Primary melanoma			Metastatic melanoma[b]	
Group	Cell line[c]	Recurrence (months)	Site	Cell line[c]
I (Early)	WM793	None (130)[d]	—	None
	WM902B	None (120)[d]	—	None
	WM35	None (150)[d]	—	None
II (Intermediate)	WM75	33	Cutis	WM373
	WM115	9	Cutis	WM165-1,WM1652
		16	Lymph node,cutis	WM239A, WM239B
		18	Cutis	WM266-1, WM266-2
	WM278	84	Cutis	WM1617
	WM98-1, WM98-2	60	Cutis	None
	WM853-2	36	Cutis	None
	WM740V[e]	9	Cutis	WM858
		11	Cutis	WM873-1, WM873-2, WM873-3
III (Advanced)	WM983A	0	Lymph nodes	WM983B, WM983C
	WM1361A	0	Cutis	WM1361B,WM1361C

[a]From Kath et al, 1990.

[b]From same patient.

[c]VGP or complex (RGP and VGP) primary melanoma lesions except WM35 (RGP).

[d]Number of months of clinical follow-up.

[e]Poor growth.

and metastatic melanoma cells. If SV40-transformed cells are supertransfected with n-*ras*, they form tumors after subcutaneous injection (L. Diamond and K. Melber, unpublished). The infection of melanocytes with an amphotropic murine sarcoma virus increases the expression of HLA-DR and GD$_3$,[76] but does not lead to growth factor independence or an infinite life span. However, spontaneous transformation and infinite life span can occur in *ras*-transjected melanocytes.[77]

Stepwise procedures can be used to select VGP primary melanoma cell variants from uncloned mass cultures that have characteristics of metastatic cells. Table 11 outlines four

in vivo and in vitro approaches used by our laboratory to obtain cell variants with invasive and metastatic properties through natural selection. The WM793 primary melanoma cell line of the early group was found after successive intravenous and subcutaneous injections in nude mice to metastasize to the lungs after subcutaneous injection.[78] The same cell line was also selected for high levels of invasiveness of the basement membrane reconstruct, 'Matrigel', and to grow independently of any exogenous growth factors.[79] The two procedures, selection of growth factor independence and invasiveness, can also be combined. We have previously shown[80,81] that melanoma

Table 8. Growth characteristics of primary and metastatic melanoma cell lines[a]

Group	Melanoma Lesion	Cell line	Population doublings per day[b]	% CFE at clonal densities	% CFE in soft agar	Tumor growth in nude mice
I. (Early)	Primary	WM793	0.29[c]	1.0[c]	7.2	s[d]
II. (Intermediate)	Primary	WM902B	0.31	1.8	6.5	s
	Metastasis	WM373[e]	0.30	9.6	29.8	r
	Primary	WM115	0.22	1.0	6.0	s
	Metastasis	WM239A[e]	0.38	3.6	9.0	r
III (Advanced)	Primary	WM983A	0.51	21.0	75.0	rr
	Metastasis	WM983B[e]	0.65	24.0	85.0	rr
	Metastasis	WM983C[e]	0.65	23.0	72.0	rr
	Primary	WM1361A	0.35	16.0	0.8	s
	Metastasis	WM1361C[e]	0.29	14.0	1.0	s

[a]From Kath et al, 1990.

[b]After seeding at high density (104/cm^2) and determined between days 1 and 8.

[c]Mean of triplicates with less than 10% standard deviation.

[d]Tumor mass after 10 weeks: s = < 0.5 g; r = 0.5 to 1.0 g; rr > 1.0 g.

[e]From same patient as primary cell line.

Table 9. Stimulation of primary and metastatic melanoma cell lines by exogenous mitogens[a]

Group	Source	Cell line	Base medium	Insulin (5 g/ml)	EGF (5 ng/ml)	Transferrin (10 mg/ml)	Combination insulin, EGF transferrin	2% FCS
							Percent increase in cell number[b]	
I (Early)	Primary	WM902B	0	50	40	0	60	460
		WM793	0	110	0	0	100	420
II (Intermediate)	Primary	WM115	0	35	0	0	30	300
	Metastatic	WM239A[c]	110	290	220	260	370	650
		WM266-4[c]	140	370	210	170	400	510
	Primary	WM75	0	0	0	0	0	590
	Metastatic	WM373[c]	120	460	190	200	400	430
		WM164	360	790	760	620	660	720
		WM852	240	820	270	310	770	880
		WM9	0	0	0	0	0	1740

[a]From Rodeck et al, 1987.
[b]Cells were seeded at 1-2 x 104/cm² on gelatin-coated plastic.
[c]From same patient.

Table 10. Characteristics of experimentally and spontaneously transformed human melanocytes

Transforming agent	Soft agar growth	Growth factor independence	Stimulation by phorbol ester	Indefinite life span	Tumorigenicity in nude mice
Ad12/SV40 hybrid virus	++[a]	++	0	++	0
SV40 T antigen gene	++	++	0	++	0
MSV (Ha-*ras*)	0	0	++	0	N.D.
SV40 T + n-*ras*	N.D.	++	0	++	++
Spontaneous (nevus)	++	0	++	0	0
Spontaneous (VGP melanoma)	++	0	0	++	++
Spontaneous (metastatic melanoma)	++	++	0	++	++

[a]++, yes; 0, no; N.D., not determined.

cells from a metastatic lesion can be selected in vitro for invasiveness and these can be metastatic in nude mice.

In vivo selected melanoma cells that metastasize in nude mice show a number of differences from the parental cells that help to clarify the various factors involved in metastasis.[80,81] Metastatic cells isolated and cultured from the lungs of nude mice grow more slowly than parental cells in the presence of serum but more rapidly in protein-free medium, and they also grow with higher colony-forming efficiency in soft agar indicating a high level of endogenous growth factor production for autocrine growth stimulation (Table 12). Metastatic cells have higher activities of tissue plasminogen activator and collagenase. Their invasion of Matrigel can be inhibited with an-

tibodies against tissue plasminogen activator.

Several approaches in the murine system have lead to malignant transformation of melanocytes. First, murine melanocytes are transfected with oncogenes or growth factor genes. Melanocytes transfected with either n-*ras* or c-*myc* are immortal and tumorigenic, those transfected with bFGF are immortal but nontumorigenic.[82-84] Second, mice transgenic for SV40 T under the tyrosinase promoter spontaneously develop tumors in pigmented cells.[85,86] Transgenic mice with overexpressed *ret* also develop melanomas (see Chapter 3—c-*ret*). Third, treatment of newborn mice with chemical carcinogenes and TPA or UV-B as promoters leads to melanoma formation (see Chapter 3—The potential role of ultraviolet light in melanoma development).

Table 11. Progression of VGP primary melanoma cells by natural selection

Type	Cell line	Stepwise selection for
In vivo	WM793	Metastasis in nude mice (s.c. to lungs and lymph nodes)
In vitro	WM75	Invasion of basement membranes
	WM793	
	WM278	
	WM902B	
	WM115	
In vitro	WM75	Growth factor independence
	WM793	
	WM278	
	WM902B	
In vitro	WM75	Independence from growth factors and high invasiveness of basement membranes
	WM793	

Table 12. In vitro characteristics of a melanoma cell line before and after selection for metastasis formation in nude mice

Characteristic	Parental cell line WM164	Metastatic variant 451Lu
Growth in serum (Population doublings in h)	48	72
Growth in protein-free medium (Population doublings in h)	221	94
Colony formation in soft agar(%)	2.0	17
In vitro invasiveness (cells/field)	9.2	25.0
Collagenase type IV (ng/ml)	0.05	0.6
Tissue plasminogen activator (mPu/mg)	8.5	25.1

REFERENCES

1. Hirobe T. Genes involved in regulating the melanocyte and melanoblast-melanocyte populations in the epidermis of newborn mouse skin. J Exp Zool 1982; 223:257-264.
2. Bennett DC, Bridges K, McKay IA. Clonal separation of mature melanocytes from premelanocytes in a diploid human cell strain: Spontaneous and induced pigmentation of premelanocytes. J Cell Sci 1985; 77:167-183.
3. Bennett DC. Differentiation in mouse melanoma cells: Initial reversibility and an on-off stochastic model. Cell 1983; 34:445-453.
4. Bennett DC. Mechanisms of differentiation in melanoma cells and melanocytes. Environ Health Persp 1989; 80:49-59.
5. Staricco RG. Amelanotic melanocytes in the outer sheath of the human hair follicle and their role in the pigmentation of regenerated epidermis. Ann NY Acad Sci 1963; 100:239-255.
6. Jimbow K, Salopek TG, Dixon WT, Searles GE, Yamada K. The epidermal melanin unit in the pathophysiology of malignant melanoma. Am J Dermatol 1991; 13:179-188.
7. Clark WH Jr, Elder DE, Guerry D IV, Epstein MN, Greene MH, Van Horn M. A study of tumor progression: The precursor lesions of superficial spreading and nodular melanoma. Hum Pathol 1984; 15:1147-1165.
8. Greene MH, Clark WH Jr, Tucker M, Elder DE, Kraemer KH, Guerry D IV, Witmer WK, Thompson J, Matozzo I, Fraser MC. Acquired precursors of cutaneous malignant melanoma. The familial dysplastic nevus syndrome. N Engl J Med 1985; 312:91-97.
9. Clark WH Jr. Human cutaneous malignant melanoma as a model for cancer. Cancer Metastasis Rev 1991; 10:83-88.
10. Clark WH Jr, Elder DE, Guerry D IV, Braitman LE, Trock BJ, Schultz D, Synnestvedt M, Halpern AC. Model predicting survival in stage I melanoma based on tumor progression. J Natl Cancer Inst 1989; 82:626-627.
11. Clark WH Jr. Tumor progression and the nature of cancer. Br J Cancer 1991; 64:631-644.
12. Elder DE, Clark WH Jr, Glenitsas R, Guerry D IV, Halpern AC. The early and intermediate precursor lesions of tumor progression in melanocytic system: Common acquired nevi and atypical (dysplastic) nevi. Sem Diagnostic Pathol, 1993.
13. Rhodes AR, Melski JW. Small congenital nevocellular nevi and the risk of cutaneous melanoma. J Pediatr 1982; 100:219-224.
14. Greene MH. Rashomon and the procrustean bed: A tale of dysplastic nevi. J Natl Cancer Inst 1991; 83:1720-1724.

15. Wayte DM, Helwig EB. Halo nevi. Cancer 1968; 22:69-89.

16. Goovaerts G, Buyssens N. Nevus cell maturation or atrophy. Am J Dermatol 1988; 10:20-27.

17. Lund HZ, Stobbe GD. The natural history of pigmented nevus: Factors of age and anatomic location. Am J Pathol 1949; 6:1117-1147.

18. Sagebiel RW. The dysplastic melanocytic nevus. J Am Acad Dermatol 1989; 20:496-501.

19. NIH Consensus Development Panel on Early Melanoma. Diagnosis and treatment of early melanoma. JAMA 1992; 268:1314-1319.

20. Clark WH Jr, Reimer RR, Greene MH, Ainsworth AA, Mastrangelo MJ. Origin of familial melanomas from heritable melanocytic lesions. Arch Dermatol 1978; 114:732-738.

21. Elder DE, Goldman SC, Greene MH, Clark WH Jr. Dysplastic nevus syndrome: A phenotypic association of sporadic cutaneous melanoma. Cancer 1980; 46:1787-1794.

22. National Institutes of Health. Precursors to malignant melanoma. National Institutes of Health, Oct 24-26, 1983. Am J Dermatol 1984; 6:169-174.

23. Elder DE, Greene MH, Guerry D IV, Kraemer KH, Clark WH Jr. The dysplastic nevus syndrome: Our definition. Am J Dermatol 1982; 4:455-460.

24. Valyi-Nagy IT, Herlyn M. Regulation of growth and phenotype of normal human melanocytes in culture. In: Nathanson L, ed. Melanoma 5, series on cancer treatment and research. Boston: Kluwer Academic Publishers, 1991:85-101.

25. Karasek M, Charlton ME. Isolation and growth of normal human skin melanocytes (abstr). Clin Res 1980; 28:570A.

26. Kitano Y. Stimulation by melanocyte stimulating hormone and dibutyryl adenosine 3', 5'-cyclic monophosphate of DNA synthesis in human melanocytes in vitro. Arch Derm Res 1976; 257:47-52.

27. Mayer TC. The control of embryonic pigment cell proliferation in culture by cyclic AMP. Dev Biol 1982; 94:509-614.

28. Wilkins LM, Szabo GC. Use of mycostatin-supplemented media to establish pure epi-dermal melanocyte culture (abstr). J Invest Dermatol 1981; 76:332A.

29. Eisinger M, Marko O. Selective proliferation of normal human melanocytes in vitro in the presence of phorbol ester and cholera toxin. Proc Natl Acad Sci USA 1982; 79:2018-2022.

30. Gilchrest BA, Vrabel MA, Flynn E, Szabo G. Selective cultivation of human melanocytes from newborn and adult epidermis. J Invest Dermatol 1984; 83:370-376.

31. Rosdahl IK, Szabo G. Mitotic activity of epidermal melanocytes in UV-irradiated mouse skin. J Invest Dermatol 1978; 70:143-148.

32. Friedman PS, Gilchrest BA. Ultraviolet radiation directly induces pigment production by cultured human melanocytes. J Cell Physiol 1987; 133:88-94.

33. Libow LF, Scheide S, DeLeo VA. Ultraviolet radiation acts as an independent mitogen for normal human melanocytes in culture. Pigment Cell Res 1988; 1:397-401.

34. Stierner U, Rosdahl I, Augustsson A, Kagedal B. UVB irradiation induces melanocyte increase in both exposed and shielded human skin. J Invest Dermatol 1989; 92:561-564.

35. Halaban R, Ghosh S, Baird A. bFGF is the putative natural growth factor for human melanocytes. In Vitro 1987; 23:47-52.

36. Halaban R, Kwon BS, Ghosh S, Delli Bovi P, Baird A. bFGF as an autocrine growth factor for human melanomas. Oncogene Res 1988; 3:177-186.

37. Halaban R. Growth factors regulating normal and malignant melanocytes. In: Nathanson L, ed. Melanoma Research: genetics, growth factors, metastases, and antigens. Boston: Kluwer Academic Publishers, 1991:19-40.

38. Funasaka Y, Boulton T, Cobb M, Yarden Y, Fan B, Lyman SD, Williams DE, Anderson DM, Zakut R, Mishima Y, Halaban R. c-Kit-Kinase induces a cascade of protein tyrosine phosphorylation in normal human melanocytes in response to mast cell growth factor and stimulates mitogen-activated protein kinase but is down-regulated in melanomas. Mol Biol Cell 1992; 3:197-209.

39. Rubin JS, Chan AM, Bottaro DP, Burgess WH, Taylor WG, Cech AC, Hirschfeld DW,

Wong J, Miki T, Finch PW, Aaronson SA. A broad spectrum human lung fibroblast-derived mitogen is a variant of hepatocyte growth factor. Proc Natl Acad Sci USA 1991; 88:415-419.

40. Halaban R, Rubin JS, Funasaka Y, Cobb M, Boulton T, Faletto D, Rosen E, Chan A, Yoko K, White W, Cook C, Moellmann G. Met and hepatocyte growth factor/scatter factor signal transduction in normal melanocytes and melanoma cells. Oncogene 1992; 7:2195-2206.

41. Rodeck U, Herlyn M, Menssen HD, Furlanetto RW, Koprowski H. Metastatic but not primary melanoma cell lines grow in vitro independently of exogenous growth factors. Int J Cancer 1987; 40:687-690.

42. Herlyn M, Rodeck U, Mancianti ML, Cardillo FM, Lang A, Ross AH, Jambrosic J, Koprowski H. Expression of melanoma-associated antigens in rapidly dividing human melanocytes in culture. Cancer Res 1987; 47:3057-3061.

43. Herlyn M, Clark WH Jr, Rodeck U, Mancianti ML, Jambrosic J, Koprowski H. Biology of tumor progression in human melanocytes. Lab Invest 1987; 56:461-474.

44. Pittelkow MR, Shipley GD. Serum-free culture of normal human melanocytes: Growth kinetics and growth factor requirements. J Cell Physiol 1989; 140:565-576.

45. Herlyn M, Mancianti ML, Jambrosic J, Bolen JB, Koprowski H. Regulatory factors that determine growth and phenotype of normal human melanocytes. Exp Cell Res 1988; 179:322-331.

46. Abdel-Malek ZA. Endocrine factors as effectors of integumental pigmentation. In: Dermatologic Clinics, Vol. 6. Philadelphia: W.B. Saunders, 1988; pp 175-184.

47. Adashi EY, Resnick CE, Svoboda ME, Van Wyk JJ. Follicle-stimulating hormone enhances somatomedin C binding to cultured rat granulosa cells. J Biol Chem 1986; 261:3923-3926.

48. Morelli JG, Norris DA. Influence of inflammatory mediators and cytokines on human melanocyte function. J Invest Dermatol 1993; 100:191S-195.

49. Medrano EE, Farooqui JZ, Boissy RE, Boissy YL, Akadiri B, Nordlund JJ. Chronic growth stimulation of human adult melanocytes by inflammatory mediators in vitro: Implications for nevus formation and initial steps in melanocyte oncogenesis. Proc. Natl. Acad. Sci. USA 1993; 90:1790-1794.

50. Morelli JG, Hake SS, Murphy RC, Norris DA. Leukotriene B$_4$-induced human melanocyte pigmentation and leukotriene C$_4$-induced human melanocyte growth are inhibited by different isoquinoline sulfonamides. J Invest Dermatol 1992; 98:55-58.

51. Fossati G, Taramelli D, Balsari A, Bogdanovich G, Andreola S, Parmiani G. Primary but not metastatic melanoma expressing DR antigens stimulate autologous lymphocytes. Int J Cancer 1984; 33:591-597.

52. Imokawa G, Yada Y, Miyagishi M. Endothelins secreted from human keratinocytes are intrinsic mitogens for human melanocytes. J Biol Chem 1992; 267:24675-24680.

53. Tomita Y, Iwamoto M, Masuda T, Tagami H. Stimulatory effect of prostaglandin E$_2$ on the configuration of normal human melanocytes in vitro. J Invest Dermatol 1987; 89:299-301.

54. Halaban R. Responses of cultured melanocytes to defined growth factors. Pigmented Cell Res (Suppl) 1988; 1:18-26.

55. McEwan MT, Parsons PG. Regulation of tyrosinase expression and activity in human melanoma cells via histamine redceptors. J Invest Dermatol (United States), 1991; 97(5):868-73.

56. Frankel TL, Mason RS, Hersey E, Posen S. The synthesis of vitamin D metabolites by human melanoma cells. J Clin Endocrinol Metab 1983; 57:627-631.

57. Bikle DD, Nemanic MK, Gee E, Elias P. 1,25-dihyroxy vitamin D$_3$ production by human keratinocytes. J Clin Invest 1986; 78:557-566.

58. Tomita Y, Torinuki W, Tagami H. Stimulation of human melanocytes by vitamin D$_3$ possibly mediates skin pigmentation after sun exposure. J Invest Dermatol 1988; 90:882-884.

59. Abdel-Malek ZA, Ross R, Trinkle L, Swope V, Pike JW, Nordlund JJ. Hormonal effects of vitamin D$_3$ on epidermal melanocytes. J Cell Physiol 1988; 136:273-280.

60. Ranson M, Posen S, Mason RS. Extracellular matrix modulates the function of human melanocytes but not melanoma cells. J Cell Physiol 1988; 136:281-288.

61. Valyi-Nagy I, Hirka G, Jensen PJ, Shih I-M, Juhasz I, Herlyn M. Undifferentiated keratinocytes control growth, morphology and antigen expression of normal melanocytes through cell-cell contact. Lab Invest, In press.

62. Herlyn M, Herlyn D, Elder DE, Bondi E, La Rossa D, Hamilton R, Sears HF, Balaban G, Guerry D IV, Clark WH Jr, Koprowski H. Phenotypic characteristics of cells derived from precursors of human melanoma. Cancer Res 1983; 43:5502-5508.

63. Herlyn M, Thurin J, Balaban G, Bennicelli JL, Herlyn D, Elder DE, Bondi E, Guerry D IV, Nowell P, Clark WH Jr, Koprowski H. Characteristics of cultured human melanocytes isolated from different stages of tumor progression. Cancer Res 1985; 45:5670-5676.

64. Mancianti ML, Herlyn M, Weil D, Jambrosic J, Rodeck U, Becker D, Diamond L, Clark WH Jr, Koprowski H. Growth and phenotypic characteristics of human nevus cells in culture. J Invest Dermatol 1988; 90:134-141.

65. Balaban G, Herlyn M, Elder DE, Bartolo R, Koprowski H, Clark WH Jr, Nowell PC. Cytogenetics of human malignant melanoma and premalignant lesions. Cancer Genet Cytogenet 1984; 11:429-439.

66. Richmond A, Fine R, Murray D, Lawson DH, Priest JH. Growth factor and cytogenetic abnormalities in cultured nevi and malignant melanomas. J Invest Dermatol 1986; 86:295-302.

67. Mancianti ML, Clark WH Jr, Hayes FA, Herlyn M. Malignant melanoma stimulants arising in congenital melanocytic nevi do not show experimental evidence for a malignant phenotype. Am J Pathol 1990; 136:817-829.

68. Mancianti ML, Györfi T, Shih I-M, Valyi-Nagy I, Levengood G, Menssen HD, Halpern AC, Elder DE, Herlyn M. Growth regulation of cultured human nevus cells. J Invest Dermatol 1993; 100:281S-287S.

69. Balaban G, Herlyn M, Elder DE, Bartolo R, Koprowski H, Clark WH Jr, Nowell PC. Cytogenetics of human malignant melanoma and premalignant lesions. Cancer Genet Cytogenet 1984; 11:429-439.

70. Balaban GB, Herlyn M, Clark WH Jr, Nowell P. Karyotypic evolution in human malignant melanoma. Cancer Genet Cytogenet 1986; 19:113-122.

71. Kath R, Rodeck U, Parmiter A, Jambrosic J, Herlyn M. Growth factor independence in vitro of primary melanoma cells from advanced but not early or intermediate lesions. Cancer Therapy and Control 1990; 1:179-191.

72. Herlyn M, Balaban G, Bennicelli J, Guerry D IV, Halaban R, Herlyn D, Elder DE, Maul GG, Steplewski Z, Nowell PC, Clark WH Jr, Koprowski H. Primary melanoma cells of the vertical growth phase: Similarities to metastatic cells. J Natl Cancer Inst 1985; 74:283-289.

73. Rodeck U, Herlyn M, Menssen HD, Furlanetto RW, Koprowski H. Metastatic but not primary melanoma cells grow in vitro independently of exogenous growth factors. Int J Cancer 1987; 40:687-690.

74. Jambrosic J, Mancianti ML, Ricciardi RP, Sela BA, Koprowski H, Herlyn M. Transformation of normal human melanocytes and non-malignant nevus cells by adenovirus 12-SV40 hybrid virus. Int J Cancer 1989; 44:1117-1123.

75. Melber K, Zhu G, Diamond L. SV40-transfected human melanocyte sensitivity to growth inhibition by the phorbolester 12-O-tetradecanoyl-phorbol-13-acetate. Cancer Res 1989; 49:3650-3655.

76. Albino AP, Houghton AN, Eisinger M, Lee JS, Kantor RRS, Oliff AI, Old LJ. Class II histocompatibility antigen expression in human melanocytes transformed by Harvey murine sarcoma virus (Ha-MSV) and Kirsten MSV retroviruses. J Exp Med 1986; 164:1710-1722.

77. Albino AP, Sozzi G, Nanus DM, Jhanwar SC, Houghton AN. Malignant transformation of human melanocytes-induction of a complete melanoma phenotype and genotype. Oncogene 1992; 7:2315-2321.

78. Juhasz I, Albelda SM, Elder DE, Murphy GF, Valyi-Nagy IT, Herlyn M. Growth and invasion of human melanomas in human skin grafted to immunodeficient mice. Am J Pathol, In press.

79. Kath R, Jambrosic J, Holland L, Rodeck U,

Herlyn M. Development of invasive and growth factor independent cell variants from primary melanomas. Cancer Res 1991; 51:2205-2211.

80. Iliopoulos D, Ernst C, Steplewski Z, Jambrosic JA, Rodeck U, Herlyn M, Clark WH Jr, Koprowski H, Herlyn D. Inhibition of metastasis of a human melanoma xenograft by monoclonal antibody to the GD2/GD3 gangliosides. J Natl Cancer Inst 1989; 81:440-444.

81. Herlyn D, Iliopoulos D, Jensen PJ, Parmiter A, Baird J, Hotta H, Ross AH, Jambrosic J, Koprowski H, Herlyn M. In vitro properties of human melanoma cells metastatic in nude mice. Cancer Res 1990; 50:2296-2302.

82. Dotto GP, Moellmann G, Ghosh S, Edwards M, Halaban R. Transformation of murine melanocytes by basic fibroblast growth factor cDNA and oncogenes and selective suppression of the transformed phenotype in a recon-stituted cutaneous environment. J Cell Biol 1989; 109:3115-3128.

83. Wilson RE, Dooley TP, Hart IR. Induction of tumorigenicity and lack of in vitro growth requirement for 12-O-tetradecanoylphorbol-13-acetate by transfection of murine melanocytes with v-Ha-*ras*. Cancer Res 1989; 49:711-716.

84. Dotto GP, Ramon Y, Cajal S, Suster S, Halaban R, Filvaroff E. Induction of different morphologic features of malignant melanoma and pigmented lesions after transformation of murine melanocytes with bFGF-cDNA and H-*ras*, *myc*, *neu*, and E1A oncogenes. Am J Pathol 1991; 138:349-358.

85. Bradl M, Klein-Szanto A, Porter S, Mintz B. Malignant melanoma in transgenic mice. Proc Natl Acad Sci USA 1991; 88:164-168.

86. Klein-Szanto A, Bradl M, Porter S, Mintz B. Melanosis and associated tumors in transgenic mice. Proc Natl Acad Sci USA 1991; 88:169-173.

CHAPTER 5

STRUCTURE AND FUNCTION OF MOLECULES EXPRESSED BY MELANOMA CELLS

The use of murine MAb led to the subsequent characterization of major antigenic systems, each consisting of several immunologically and biologically distinct structures [reviewed in refs. 1-6]. As illustrated in Figure 9, a variety of proteins and carbohydrates are expressed by melanoma cells. Without exception, these proteins and carbohydrates can also be found on some normal cells of other cell lineages. They are, therefore, not tumor-specific, but tumor-associated because of qualitative or quantitative differences in expression between normal melanocytes and melanoma cells.

In the following, melanoma-associated antigens are grouped according to their biological functions, since recent studies on functions of melanoma-associated antigens provide information on approaches for diagnosis and therapy, and on understanding development and progression of melanoma. This classification can now be attempted because of better knowledge of the biochemical and molecular structures of melanoma-associated antigens. However, these tumor-associated antigens may have multiple functions, and the division into functional groups is often arbitrary and will need future revisions.

Heterogeneity of antigen expression between malignant cells within one lesion and between lesions of the same or different patients is a significant factor in studies of tumor-associated antigens. Heterogeneity may vary between different antigens and may depend on the regulation of expression by tumor- or host-derived factors. Some of the factors regulating the expression of tumor-associated antigens have been reviewed.[7]

Part of the information on the expression of melanoma-associated antigens is derived from cultured cells, and part is obtained from in situ studies. Many differences in the expression of antigens exist between normal melanocytes in vitro and in situ.[8] These differences may relate to the expression of cell surface molecules or to the expression of secreted cytoplasmic proteins. In melanoma, on the other hand, differences between cells in vitro and in vivo are uncommon and may only be quantitative. Thus, comparisons between cells of different stages of tumor progression are done predominantly on tissue sections and not on cultured cells, unless use of the latter is unavoidable.

ADHESION RECEPTORS AND THEIR LIGANDS

Cell surface antigens involved in adhesion may mediate cell-matrix or cell-cell interactions. Many adhesion receptors may exert multiple functions through their involvement in cell-cell and cell-substrate contacts and in other signalling events.

INTEGRINS

Melanoma cells express a large number of different integrins, and integrin expression is higher on metastatic melanoma cells than on primary melanoma cells. This upregulation of integrin expression with tumor progression is highly "melanoma-associated", since tumors derived from epithelial cells often suppress the expression of adhesion receptors.[9] The integrin receptor family, as summarized in Table 13, has vastly increased over the last years and comprises at least 20 pro-

teins.[10] Each integrin is a heterodimer consisting of an α subunit that is non-covalently associated with a β subunit. The receptor complex spans the plasma membrane, linking the internal cytoskeletal network with the extracellular matrix. Specificity for ligand binding is determined by the particular association of α and β subunits. The integrins are divided into subfamilies, each defined by a common β subunit.[10,11] Antibodies to integrins inhibit attachment of tumor and normal cells to substrate. As listed in Table 13, many integrins are expressed on melanoma cells.[12] Expression increases in more advanced tumors. Of the β_1 subfamily, melanoma cells express α_1 through α_7[12,13] and α_v,[14] which include receptors for laminin, fibronectin, and collagens. α_v can also associate with several other β subunits, including β_3, β_5, β_6, and β_8. Except β_8, all $\alpha_v\beta$ combinations have been found on melanoma cells.

Of the β_1 subfamily, $\alpha_2\beta_1$ expression distinguishes invasive from noninvasive melanoma

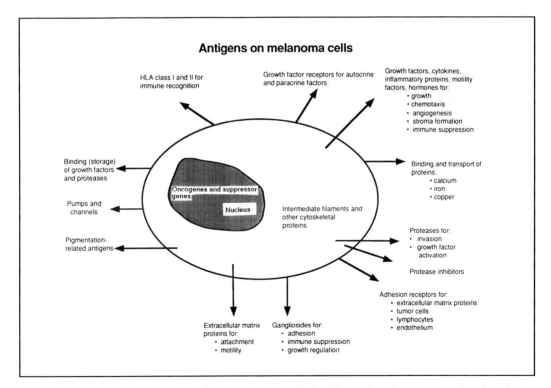

Fig. 9. Schematic illustration of the expression and shedding of melanoma-associated antigens. Pigmentation-related antigens, cytoskeletal proteins, extracellular matrix proteins, and intermediate filaments are not expressed on the cell surface. All others may be at least temporarily expressed.

Table 13. The integrin receptor family and its expression on melanoma cells[a]

Subunits		Ligands and counter receptors	Binding site	Expression on melanoma cells[b]	References[c]
b1	a1	Collagens, laminin		++[c]	11,21
	a2	Collagens, laminin	DGEA	+	
	a3	Fibronectin, laminin, collagens	RGD ±?	++	11,15
	a4	Fibronectin (V25), VCAM-1	EILDV	++	11,22
	a5	Fibronectin (RGD)	RGD	±	9,11
	a6	Laminin		++	11
	a7	Laminin		++	13
	a8	?		?	
	av	Vitronectin, fibronectin (?)	RGD	++	23
b2	aL	ICAM-1, ICAM-2		?	
	aM	C3b component of complement (inactivated)	GPRP	?	
b3	aIIb	Fibrinogen, fibronectin, von Willebrand factor, vitronectin, thrombospondin	RGD, KQAGDV	+	14
	av	Vitronectin, fibrinogen, von Willebrand factor, thrombospondin, fibronectin, osteopontin, collagen	RGD	++	11,24
b4	a6	Laminin ?		−	
b5	av	Vitronectin	RGD	++?	
b6	av	Fibronectin	RGD	++?	
b7	a4	Fibronectin (V25) VCAM-1	EILDV	?	
	aIEL	?		?	
b8	av	?	?	?	

[a]Modified from Hynes, 1992.

[b]++, strong; +, intermediate; -, negative; ?, no information available.

[c]For expression on melanoma cells only.

cells.[15,16] $\alpha_4\beta_1$ is of interest because the ligand for this receptor is not only fibronectin but also VCAM-1 (INCMA-110), which is found on IL-1-stimulated endothelial cells.[17] The $\alpha_4\beta_1$-VCAM-1 association may stimulate attachment of melanoma cells to the endothelium, thereby enhancing the arrest of circulating melanoma cells in small capillaries.

The β_3 subunit is strikingly upregulated in melanoma progression.[12] This overexpression is clearly associated with the invasive nature of VGP primary melanoma lesions (Table 14). Whereas none of 12 RGP primary melanoma lesions expressed this subunit, 8 of 10 VGP and all of 11 metastatic melanomas expressed it. The $\alpha_v\beta_3$ integrin can bind a large number of extracellular matrix proteins including vitronectin, fibrinogen, von Willebrand factor, thrombospondin, fibronectin, osteopontin, and collagen (Table 13). All ligands contain the RGD amino acid sequence and bind $\alpha_v\beta_3$ apparently through this association. However, melanoma cells can also use the $\alpha_v\beta_3$ integrin to matrix proteins such as fibrinogen in attaching to alternative adhesive sites that are independent of the RGD sequence.[18] On the other hand, the $\alpha_v\beta_3$ appears to act in concert with the fibronectin receptor $\alpha_5\beta_1$ to attach to fibronectin as a substrate.[19] $\alpha_v\beta_3$ plays a major role in invasion and metastasis; treatment of A375 melanoma cells

with polyclonal or monoclonal antibodies to $\alpha_v\beta_3$ stimulated invasion of melanoma cells through a reconstructed basement membrane.[20] Similar invasion-enhancing effects were also seen when cells were incubated with vitronectin. Metastatic melanoma cells adhere to sections of lymph nodes more readily than the parental cells.[25] This adhesion apparently occurs through an $\alpha_v\beta_3$-RGD mechanism.

The activation of integrins through signal transduction and secondary signalling due to this activation are still poorly understood. Apparently, the receptor undergoes conformational changes between at least two states: inactive and active.[10] Only active receptors can bind the ligand. Changes can occur through regulation of affinity and conformation of the receptor from the cell interior, and through intracellular events triggered by ligand occupation of the receptors. Whether and how such signaling occurs in melanoma cells requires investigation because adhesion antagonists may provide a new therapeutic approach to prevent metastasis formation.

NON-INTEGRIN MATRIX ADHESION RECEPTORS

Of the non-integrin adhesion receptors, at least two, possibly three, are expressed on melanoma cells. One is the 67 kDa laminin

Table 14. Expression of the β_3 subunit of the vitronectin receptor in melanocytic tissues[a]

Tissue	Specimens expressing β_3 subunit/total tested
Skin (melanocyte)	0/8
Nevus	0/9
RGP primary melanoma	0/12
VGP primary melanoma	8/10
Metastatic melanoma	11/11

[a]All assays were done on frozen sections with monoclonal antibody specific for the subunit.

receptor which interacts with the YIGSR sequence in the β_1 chain of laminin. Expression of this receptor correlates with metastasis which can be inhibited by the YIGSR amino acid peptide.[26-28] A peptide (peptide 6) from the cDNA sequence for a 33 kDa protein related to the 67 kDa laminin receptor specifically inhibited binding of laminin to heparin and sulfatide.[29] However, this inhibition may be due to the inhibition of another heparin-binding protein with the same sulfated ligands rather than specific inhibition of laminin binding to the 67 kDa receptor. The second is the cell surface glycoprotein CD44, which is expressed on many cell types. By binding to hyaluronic acid, it plays a role in cell-matrix interactions, but it can also self-associate in cell-cell binding.[30-32] Human CD44 has recently been shown to increase the tumorigenic potential of lymphoma cells,[31] and the murine homolog of CD44 can confer metastatic potential to epithelial tumor cell lines.[33,34] A recently identified splice variant of the homing receptor CD44 (the Hermes antigen) was shown to confer metastatic capability to non-malignant rat colon tumor cells.[34,35] The CD44 variant cDNA was cloned using a MAb that detects a protein epitope present only on colon carcinoma cell lines with high, metastatic potential.[33] The epitope consists of 162 amino acids inserted into the extracellular domain of CD44 by alternative RNA splicing. Overexpression of the CD44 variant in non-metastasizing cells by cDNA transfection resulted in full metastatic potential.[34] Some clues to the mechanism by which the variant CD44 promotes metastasis come from the study of the normal function of CD44 proteins. CD44 is a 80-90 kDa transmembrane glycoprotein that bears homologies in its extracellular domain to cartilage link and proteoglycan core proteins.

In melanoma, CD44 is highly expressed and expression correlates with in vitro migration and invasiveness on hyaluronate substrates.[36] These results confirm studies in the murine system demonstrating that invading tumor cells stimulate production of hyaluronate by host tissue stroma[37,38] and stromal cells.[38,39] The presence of a loose coat of hyaluronic acid around the most aggressive murine melanoma

cells appears permissive for in vivo invasiveness,[39] and locomotion of transformed cells has been shown to be related to the presence of hyaluronic acid.[40]

Chondroitin sulfate proteoglycan (see Chapter 5.) which is strongly expressed by melanoma cells, is possibly another adhesion receptor on melanoma cells.[41] This molecule appears to modify the function and/or activity of $\alpha_4\beta_1$ on melanoma cells due to the close proximity of the two receptors.

EXTRACELLULAR MATRIX PROTEINS

The basement membrane zone (BMZ) separates the epidermis from dermis in normal skin. Since the disorganization of the BMZ plays an important part in melanoma development and progression,[42] it is briefly described here.

The BMZ in normal skin contains: the hemidesmosome, a region of dense plaque and keratin filaments; the lower portion of the basal cells; the lamina lucida (rara) and lamina densa (basal lamina); and sub-basement membrane fibrous elements including anchoring filaments, filaments of type VII collagen between the basal cell hemidesmosomes, and the upper portion of the dermis.[43,44] A number of proteins form the lamina lucida and lamina densa of the dermal-epidermal BMZ. The lamina lucida is comprised primarily of laminin, but also contains fibronectin, tenascin, bullous pemphigoid antigen, cicatricial pemphigoid antigen, and the antigens AA3, GB3, 19-DEJ-1, and 160 kDa antigen.[45-48] Major components of the lamina densa include type IV collagen, which is solely associated with the basement membrane, entactin (nidogen), and heparan sulfate proteoglycan; minor components include epidermolysis bullosa acquisita antigen, chondroitin sulfate proteoglycan, and the KF-1, LDA-1, and LH7.2 antigens.[43,46] Thrombospondin has also been found at the dermal-epidermal junction.[49] Interactions among the various proteins enable the BMZ to act as a functionally integrated unit.[44,50-52] Variations in the location of these proteins can be noted in different tissues.[44]

Epidermal melanocytes are present within the basal cell layer in contact with the dermal-epidermal basement membrane, although melanocytes can be found in a suprabasilar locale.[54,55] On the melanocyte basal surface, both hemidesmosome-like structures and anchoring filaments are present;[56] however, a less dense and thinner basement membrane with a decreased quantity of anchoring fibrils is found in contact with melanocytes in comparison to keratinocytes.[57] In addition, the C-terminal portion of type VII collagen, epidermolysis bullosa acquisita antigen, appears to be absent in the BMZ in contact with melanocytes.[57] Indirect immunofluorescence analysis indicated the production of type IV collagen, laminin, heparan sulfate proteoglycan, and fibronectin by adult but not newborn melanocytes in vitro.[56,58] Melanocytes are very adherent to laminin and fibronectin, and most neural crest cells preferentially move toward these proteins.[59] While melanocytes can spread, proliferate and remain functionally active on a basement membrane, they cannot penetrate this structure.[53,59]

Passage of melanocytes through the basement membrane of the epidermis to the papillary dermis is associated with the formation of nevi. Despite this passage into the dermal portion of the skin, individual nevus cells or cell clusters are surrounded by a basement membrane and are separated from the dermis.[60] However, the basement membrane surrounding nevus cells lacks bullous pemphigoid antigen and anchoring fibrils of type VII collagen.[57,58] Type VII collagen is restricted to the dermal-epidermal junction, where it connects basal cells to plaques in the dermis and promotes a fusion-like attachment; thus, antibody staining for type VII collagen can differentiate epidermal and nevus basement membranes.[57] Areas of discontinuity in the basement membrane are found in regions of lymphocytic infiltrates; this is most evident in halo nevi at the border of nevus cells in which an intense lymphocytic infiltrate is seen.[60] Basement membrane staining is not found between keratinocytes and intraepidermal nevi.[60] In vitro, nevus cells produce type IV collagen, laminin, heparan sulfate proteoglycan, and fibronectin.[58]

Basement membrane discontinuity is noted in the junctional region of malignant melanoma, especially in regions of regression.[60] A basement membrane is not associated with tumor cells in the deeper dermal region.[57] While laminin is produced by malignant melanoma in the dermis, type IV collagen is decreased and almost no entactin is identified.[57] This correlates with the findings that laminin increases invasion and metastatic activity. Cells adherent to laminin are more tumorigenic than parental cells, and laminin induces the secretion of collagenase type IV.

Of all the extracellular matrix proteins, secretion of fibronectin and tenascin has been studied most extensively. Whereas secretion of fibronectin by melanoma cells has been known for a long time, secretion of tenascin has only recently been detected with MAb.[63,64] Tenascin is an extracellular matrix protein that appears to have variable effects on adhesion of cells in different tissues; it may not mediate cell adhesion, but may inhibit cell attachment to other extracellular matrix proteins, including fibronectin.[65] Tenascin, also known as hexabrachion, myotendinous antigen, glioma mesenchymal matrix antigen, T1 glycoprotein, cytoactin, and pg 150/225 is a 320 kDa, six-armed structure that is present in dense connective tissue with an oncofetal predominance.[63,65] While tenascin is produced at various times and locations during embryonic development, it is generally absent from normal tissues, but can be found during wound healing and in the lamina lucida.[45,63] Gliomas, melanomas, and stromal cells of epithelial tumors such as breast carcinomas produce tenascin constitutively.[63,66]

Increased secretion of tenascin parallels tumor progression of melanocytes in vitro; normal melanocytes secreted little or no tenascin, while metastatic melanomas produced the highest quantities (1mg/ml).[63] Increased expression of tenascin has also been associated with tumor thickness,[64] and patients with high tumor burden show increased levels of circulating tenascin in serum.[63] TGF-β increases tenascin secretion by melanoma, although addition of TGF-β to culture medium did not induce tenascin secretion in cells that do not normally secrete it.[66-68] Regardless of whether or not melanoma cells produced tenascin, the cells could not adhere to it (Table 15). Thus, one role for tenascin might be to facilitate detachment of melanoma cells (from fibronectin) for motility during invasion. These results are surprising since tenascin contains the RGD sequence of fibronectin. It appears, however, that the sequence is hidden in the folded protein and that melanoma cells lack any receptors for the adhesive sites present on tenascin.

Fibronectin contains a tripeptide that is found in platelet adhesion with the extracellular matrix proteins fibronectin, fibrinogen, laminin, osteopontin, thrombospondin, type I collagen, vitronectin, and von Willebrand factor.[69] RGD synthetic peptides can promote cell attachment, inhibit binding to RGD-containing proteins, and inhibit the formation of metastases.[69] RGD-containing peptides from snake venom, so-called anti-integrins, can inhibit adhesion of melanoma cells to fibronectin, laminin, and fibrinogen, and can inhibit lung metastasis formation.[70]

The YIGSR peptides derived from the β_1 chain of laminin can inhibit migration of cells to laminin, bind to the non-integrin laminin-binding receptor (67 kDa) and decrease lung metastasis formation of murine melanoma cells.[61,71-73] However, a 19 amino acid synthetic peptide, SIKVAV derived from the laminin α chain can increase the number of lung metastases when injected together with B16F10 murine melanoma cells.[62] When YIGSR-negative or -positive binding B16F10 cell lines were selected,[74] only the YIGSR-positive variants produced rapidly growing tumors after subcutaneous injection, and twice as many lung colonies as the parental cells after intravenous injection. The data with these variants suggest that interactions of melanoma cells with the YIGSR site on laminin are probably important for both colony formation in a target organ (lung) and subsequent tumor growth, while the SIKVAV-containing site on laminin may be more important for tumor growth. Whereas laminin fragments can increase the number of metastases, a heparin binding fragment of fibronectin decreases the number of metastases when compared to intact fibronectin.[75,76] The adhesive sites on

Table 15. Attachment of melanoma cells to extracellular matrix proteins which are also secreted by the melanoma cells.

Matrix protein	% melanoma cells attaching[a] (± SD)
Fibronectin[b]	42 ± 6.3
Tenascin[b]	<0.1 ± <0.01
Laminin	29 ± 26
Collagen type-IV	33 ± 5.2
Vitronectin	Not done
4% BSA control	0.7 ± <0.01

From Herlyn et al 1991.
[a]After 30 min.
[b]Up to 1 mg/ml secreted by cultures.

laminin and its several receptors are currently under intense investigation in several laboratories. McCarthy, Furcht and Skubitz and collaborators have defined additional sequences on laminin that could be important for melanoma invasion and growth.[77-79] These investigators have also defined new sequences on collagen type IV which are involved in adhesion.[80,81] Finally, heparin- and sulfatide-binding peptides from the type I repeats of human thrombospondin promote melanoma cell adhesion.[82] These studies should yield new and important insight into the role of the BMZ in melanoma progression.

CELL-CELL ADHESION MOLECULES

Most melanoma-associated antigens that belong to the group of cell-cell adhesion molecules are members of the immunoglobulin superfamily[83] of cell adhesion molecules (CAM) (Table 16). Adhesive interactions mediated by CAMs allow cells to sort into groups and form complex structures, and as such are of critical importance in organogenesis and tissue reconstruction. CAMs not only allow adhesion between cells, but also act as links in cell-cell signalling for growth and differentiation.[84] ICAM-1 and MUC18 of the immunoglobulin superfamily are the most highly expressed melanoma-associated antigens. Both genes have been extensively characterized in melanoma by Johnson and colleagues.[85-87] Both are markers of tumor expression and their expression on melanomas correlates with poor prognosis.

ICAM-1 (intercellular adhesion molecule-1 [CD54]) with its counter receptor LFA-1 (lymphocyte function-associated antigen-1 [CD11a]) are involved in antigen-restricted and antigen-independent immune cell contacts that are required for the preservation of an effective immune response.[84] Similar functions have also been reported for LFA-3 (CD58) and its counter receptor LFA-2 (CD-2).[84] The percentage of ICAM-1 positive cells in melanomas increases with tumor thickness[87,88] and is higher in metastatic than in

Table 16. Adhesion molecules of the immunoglobulin superfamily expressed by melanoma cells

CAM[a]	Ig domains	Ligand	Demonstrated adhesion	Reference
ICAM-1 (CD54)	5	LFA-1	Yes	109
MUC18	5	?	No	99
LFA-3 (CD58)	2	LFA-2/CD2	Yes	108
N-CAM	5	Homotypic, heparan sulfate	Yes	87,88
L-1	6	Homotypic	Yes	107
VCAM-1 (INCAM 110)	6	$\alpha_4\beta_1$ (VLA-4)	Yes	108,110
B1.1 epitope of	7/3	Homotypic and	Yes	111,112
CEA/NCA		NCA/CEA		

[a]MHC I and II are also expressed by melanoma cells, but not listed. They contain one immunoglobulin domain and bind to the T cell receptor.

primary lesions.[89] In addition, a circulating form of ICAM-1 has been recently identified[90] that is increased in the serum of melanoma patients[91] and that correlates with the clinical progression of the disease.[92] Interferon-γ and TNF-α are potent upregulators of ICAM-1 expression on a variety of cells including melanoma.[93]

ICAM-1 and LFA-3 on melanoma cells play a role in the interaction of the malignant cells with natural killer (NK) cells, lymphocyte-activated killer (LAK) cells and tumor-infiltrating lymphocytes; antibodies to ICAM-1 and LFA-3 inhibit tumor cell lysis by cytotoxic cells.[94,95] Similarly, soluble ICAM-1 can inhibit lysis of melanoma cells by NK cells,[94,96] suggesting that the soluble receptor acts as an antagonist for tumor-host adhesions.

The functional role of MUC18 in melanoma progression is less clear because the ligand for this 113 kDa molecule has not yet been identified.[97] MUC18 is remarkably specific, being present on most melanomas but not on any other tumors. Expression of MUC18 correlates with tumor thickness.[98] Expression is first seen when melanomas reach 1 mm in thickness. Of normal cells in situ, MUC18 is found only on smooth muscle cells.[97] However, antibody A32 to the MUC18 antigen also reacts with endothelial cells [I-M Shi et al, in preparation].

Sequencing revealed that MUC18, like ICAM-1 and N-CAM (neural cell adhesion molecule) has five Ig domains.[99] Preliminary evidence from our laboratory with MAb A32 suggests that the MUC18 antigen is involved in homotypic interactions. Expression of MUC18 on melanocytes and nevus cells is downregulated by undifferentiated keratinocytes; differentiated keratinocytes or fibroblasts have no effect on MUC18-expressing melanocytes or nevus cells.

Of the other members of the immunoglobulin supergene family found on melanoma cells (Table 16), N-CAM is the most prominent. N-CAM was the first intercellular adhesion molecule to be isolated, characterized, and cloned.[100,101] Although it was originally identified in neural tissues, N-CAM is now known to be broadly expressed during embryonic development and probably plays an important role in directed cell-cell interaction in many different tissues. N-CAM is encoded by a single gene, but due to differential mRNA splicing, it exists in a variety of isoforms ranging from 115 kDa to 140 kDa in apparent molecular mass.[102] N-CAM is found only in the minority of melanoma in vitro[102] and in situ.[103] Its function in the melanocyte cell system is not known. It might be involved in homotypic interactions but, since it can also bind to heparan sulfate, cell-matrix interactions through N-CAM are also possible.

The L1 adhesion molecule is also neuron-specific, and is expressed on a variety of neuroectodermal tumors,[105] including melanoma.[106] However, expression and function of human L1[107] has not been extensively studied. V-CAM-1, the ligand for $\alpha_4\beta_1$, is expressed on a few primary melanomas and expression is decreased in metastases.[104] V-CAM-1 is also expressed by nevus cells and is upregulated on melanoma by TNF-α.[108]

GANGLIOSIDES

Gangliosides are acid glycoconjugates. MAbs produced in several laboratories have defined at least five different gangliosides (Table 17): GM$_3$,[113-115] GD$_2$,[116-120] GD$_3$,[117,121-124] GM$_2$,[125] and 9-O-acetyl GD$_3$.[126-128] Many of the antibodies not only define a single ganglioside, but crossreact with others, most notably with GQ1b and GD1b.[129] Crossreactivity also varies with affinity of the antibodies. Gangliosides have different surface accessibility to antibodies, depending on total ganglioside composition of cells.[130] Expression can also depend on the micro-environment. Cultured melanoma cells have more GD$_2$ than cells in tissues, which have relatively more GD$_3$.[131] With progression, melanoma cells shift in expression from GM$_3$ towards higher GD$_3$. GD$_2$ is the most highly melanoma-associated ganglioside because it is only expressed on VGP primary and metastatic melanomas.[132] For antigen detection by MAb cultured melanoma cells must be removed mechanically or enzymatically from substrate, because gangliosides are mostly found on the substrate-adhering side of cells.

GD$_2$ and GD$_3$ are found in adhesion plaques of melanoma cells, concentrated at the site of cell-matrix interactions and on the cell surfaces.[133] Addition of exogenous gangliosides can inhibit attachment of cells to fibronectin.[133] MAbs to GD$_2$/GD$_3$ can inhibit adhesion of melanoma cells to substrate invasion through Matrigel in vitro and metastasis formation of melanomas in nude mice from a subcutaneous injection site.[133]

In addition to a role in adhesion, gangliosides may have other functions. MAb to gangliosides can stimulate lymphocytes,[134,135] apparently suppressor cells. Gangliosides can also stimulate astroglial cell proliferation,[136] suggesting that they may have a direct effect on cell proliferation.

MAJOR HISTOCOMPATIBILITY ANTIGENS

The cellular immune response to tumors requires presentation of tumor antigens to T lymphocytes. HLA molecules are required for antigen presentation, therefore one way for tumors to escape the immune response is to regulate the expression of HLA antigens.

The HLA antigens are encoded within the major histocompatibility locus on chromosome 6, a gene region that includes class I (HLA-A, -B, -C) antigens and class II (HLA-DP, -DR, and -DQ) antigens. Melanoma cells express both the class I and II products, and class II antigens appear mostly on melanoma cells that express class I antigens. Analysis of melanoma cell lines and melanocytes indicates a high degree of modulation of expression during progression[139,141-143] including a reduction or loss of HLA class I antigens and the appearance of HLA class II antigens. Neither finding is unique to melanoma, both are observed in many other malignancies. However, the frequency of the appearance of HLA class II antigens is higher in melanoma than in other neoplasms. HLA-B appears to be frequently downregulated on melanoma cells when compared to HLA-A or -C [F. Marincola, personal communication]. The role of transformation in regulating HLA expression has been confirmed in vitro experiments[144] and formation of human cultured melanocytes by the v-*ras* oncogene leads to induction of HLA class II antigens.[145]

Loss of expression of class I antigens occurs in the primary lesion, no difference is observed in the frequency of loss of HLA class I antigens between primary and metastatic lesions. Loss of class I expression may offer

Table 17. Major gangliosides expressed by melanocytic cells

Ganglioside	Expression[a]			
	Melanocyte	Nevus	Primary melanoma	Mestastic melanoma
GM3	+++	+++	+++	++
GM2	—	+	++	++
GD2	—	—	++	++
GD3	±	+	+++	++++
9-O-acetyl GD3	—	+	++	++

[a]Expression is estimated + → ++++ using MAb to gangliosides; - no expression.

distinct advantages to subpopulations of tumor cells allowing escape from a cellular immune response against the tumor. Although loss of HLA expression might provide a selective advantage, there is evidence of an associated increase in susceptibility to lysis by NK cells. On the other hand, class II antigens are expressed at a higher frequency in metastases than in primary lesions. In primary lesions, the level of expression of HLA class II antigens correlates with the depth of invasion. Thus, expression of class II antigens may offer a selective advantage to the tumor.

HLA-A2 antigen appears to be important for tumor cell recognition by autologous T lymphocytes.[146] Loss of HLA-A2 antigen expression in melanoma cells diminishes immunological recognition by T cells.[147] Transfection of HLA-A2 into antigen-negative cells restores lysability of melanoma cells. HLA class I antigens also regulate susceptibility of target cells to NK cell lysis; their upregulation reduces the susceptibility to such lysis.[148]

Cytokines can regulate the expression of HLA antigens. Interferon-γ and tumor necrosis factor-α are particularly effective in inducing HLA expression. Because T lymphocytes are the known source of interferon-γ, it is interesting that there is a relationship between expression of HLA class II antigens in primary melanoma lesions and the degree of T lymphocyte infiltration.

HLA class II antigens on primary melanoma cells, unlike those on metastatic melanomas, appear to be involved in the cell-mediated immune response. Melanoma cell lines from early malignant lesions stimulate autologous T cells to undergo blastogenesis when co-cultured in vitro.[149-151] Class II antigen expressing primary melanoma cells can function as antigen-presenting cells.[152]

GROWTH FACTORS, CYTOKINES, AND THEIR RECEPTORS

Human tumor cells produce growth factors constitutively, i.e., cultured malignant cells synthesize various ligands in the absence of any exogenous mitogens.[153] Normal cells, on the other hand, require prior stimulation by exogenous factors, and many including

melanocytes, have a reduced capacity to synthesize growth factors.[154,155] Growth factor responsiveness and synthesis by cultured normal human melanocytes, nonmalignant nevus cells, and primary and metastatic melanoma cells reflect the stage of tumor progression better than most other currently known markers.[156]

A particular factor is considered to be autocrine if all of the following criteria are met: 1) the growth factor protein is produced; 2) the receptor is expressed; and 3) suitable antagonists inhibit proliferation of the producing cell. Growth factor antagonists are a wide range of agents with variable specificity for individual growth factors. This discussion is confined to antagonists with well defined specificities; neutralizing antibodies to growth factors, antibodies that bind to and inhibit activation of growth factor receptors, and antisense oligonucleotides that presumably interrupt translation of growth factor genes in a sequence-specific manner. Furthermore, we do not consider the possibility that the cell producing a factor for autocrine stimulation should respond to this factor after it is added to the medium, since tumor cells responds variably to exogenous growth factors, depending on the media used prior to growth experiments, and they may produce growth factors in amounts already sufficient to induce maximum stimulation.

Melanoma cells express a large number of different growth factors and cytokines (Table 18), and a variety of receptors for these molecules (Table 19). In a few instances, receptor expression and ligand production are concomitant, suggesting possible autocrine pathways.[154-156] Some cell lines produce a variety of growth factors and cytokines constitutively (Table 20). These growth factors and cytokines might also be used by melanomas for paracrine effects on endothelial cells, fibroblasts, or macrophages (Table 21). Cytokines such as IL-1 produced by melanoma cells or stromal cells, may activate the production of cytokines in the same or other cells (Table 22).

Growth factor and cytokine expression by melanoma cells has been detected using different techniques: a) reverse transcriptase-polymerase chain reaction (RT-PCR) when mRNA is not abundantly present and when a large number of factors must be screened; b) conventional Northern blotting for mRNA expression; and c) protein expression using biochemical, biological, and immunological techniques. The conditions under which cells have been tested also differ widely: a) cells cultured in the presence of serum, i.e., some of the activity may be serum-induced; b) cells cultured in the absence of any exogenous mitogens to test for constitutively activated factors only; and c) in situ hybridization for mRNA expression in tissues or immunohistochemistry with antibodies to specific growth factors. Large numbers of factors have been screened,[157-161] but not all factors listed in Table 18 have been investigated by all approaches. Studies involving RT-PCR[159,161] provide the least information on the role of a given growth factor because it is unclear whether the proteins are actually expressed.

bFGF

In the melanocyte system, bFGF plays a central role as growth regulator. Normal melanocytes depend for growth and survival on the supplementation of culture medium with bFGF, whereas growth of primary and metastatic melanoma cells is bFGF independent. Nevus cells represent an intermediate stage with reduced dependence on exogenous bFGF. The independence of melanoma cells from exogenous bFGF is apparently due to autocrine growth stimulation by endogenous bFGF. All melanoma cell lines tested in our laboratory and by others express bFGF mRNA and the protein, whereas melanocytes do not[157,159,162-164] (Table 18). Inhibition of bFGF synthesis by antisense deoxyoligonucleotides suppressed melanoma cell growth in monolayer and soft agar.[162] Similarly, introduction of antibodies to bFGF into the cytoplasm inhibited melanoma cell growth.[163]

Human bFGF belongs to a family of polypeptide growth factors that includes acidic FGF,[165] the *int-2*[166] and K-*fgf/hst*[167] gene products, FGF-5,[168] FGF-6,[169] and keratinocyte growth factor (KGF). The human bFGF gene, located on chromosome 4, consists of three exons and two introns spanning at least 38 kb[170] and is transcribed into three mRNA

species of approximately 7.0, 3.7, and 1.4 kb. Analysis of human bFGF cDNA clones has revealed that bFGF is a 154-amino acid protein composed of a single polypeptide chain. Interestingly, it lacks a signal peptide that would facilitate its secretion via conventional exocytosis.[171] The common denominator of FGF family members is their high-affinity binding to heparin.[172] In addition, the factors share a similar gene structure and display extensive sequence conservation in a core region of approximately 120 amino acids. Crystallographic studies have shown that the three-dimensional structures of bovine aFGF and human bFGF are very similar.[173]

bFGF is localized in situ in a variety of normal human tissues with a predominance in endothelium, muscle, and the central nervous system.[174,175] In malignant lesions, bFGF has been found in gliomas,[176,177] and melanomas,[178] confirming studies on cultured cells. In our studies on nonmalignant nevi, we have found bFGF mRNA expressed in nevus cells within junctional areas between epidermis and dermis,[179] suggesting that bFGF expression correlates with migration of nevus cells through the basement membrane zone.

Besides its role in autocrine growth stimulation in melanoma,[162,163] glioma,[180] and adrenal carcinoma,[181] bFGF can have additional functions that are essential for tumor proliferation and dissemination, e.g., stimulation of angiogenesis, stroma formation, and invasion (Table 21). The different biological activities of bFGF have been studied mostly in normal cells and a direct role for tumor-derived bFGF in any of these paracrine functions is as yet hypothetical. However, melanoma-derived bFGF can be recovered from the extracellular matrix. bFGF is angiogenic through its attraction and growth stimulation of endothelial cells,[182,183] and it is mitogenic for fibroblasts and keratinocytes [reviewed in ref. 184]. In the extracellular matrix, bFGF is bound to heparan sulfate proteoglycan and can be released by the proteolytic enzymes plasmin or heparanase.[185] Soluble extracellular complexes of bFGF with heparan sulfate proteoglycan are biologically active[186] and may contribute to the effect of bFGF not only on producer cells but also on other cells

Table 18. Growth factors and cytokines produced by melanoma cells

Factors	% of positive cell lines[a]	Comments
bFGF	>90	Constitutive expression
K-*fgf/hst**	10	
int-2	>80	
KGF*	>90	
PDGF-α	>80	No receptor expressed
PDGF-β	~20	No receptor expressed
TGF-β_1	>90	Constitutive expression
TGF-β_2*	~50	Melanomas only
TGF-β_3*	>90	Also in melanocytes
TGF-α	~50	Constitutive expression
pleiotrophin	~80	No receptor ?
Steel (SCF)*	>80	Decreased receptor
IL-1α	~35	Stimulated by α–, β–, γ–MSH
IL-1β	60	Stimulated by α–, β–, γ-MSH
IL-6[b]	>80	Stimulated by α–, β–, γ-MSH
IL-7*	>80	
IL-8	30-100	Stimulated by serum
MGSA/gro	30-100	Stimulated by serum
LIF[b]*	>80	
IL-10*	~70	
NKSF-L (IL-12)*	15	NKSF-H not expressed
GM-CSF	~50	
G-CSF	~50	
Rantes*	~90	
TNF-α	~30	Stimulated by α–, β–, γ-MSH
IFN-β*	~10	
α-MSH	>80	
γIP-10		γ-interferon-induced

[a]Summaries (estimates) from studies in different laboratories. (Rodeck et al, 1991; Albino et al, 1991; Colombo et al, 1992; Mattei et al, submitted).
[b]Share same gp130 as part of receptor.
*Detection by RT-PCR only.

Table 19. Expression of receptors for growth factors and cytokines by melanoma cells

Receptor	Primary ligand	Other ligands binding same receptor
EGFR	EGF	TGF-α, amphiregulin, HB-EGF, crypto
IGF-IR	IGF-I	Insulin
FGFR-1	bFGF	aFGF, *int*-2, FGF-5, FGF-6
c-kit	SCF (steel)	-
met	SF	-
NGFR[a]	NGF	-
Transferrin R	Transferrin	-
TGF-βR1	TGF-β_2	TGF-β_2, TGF-β_3
MSH	α-MSH	β-MSH, ACTH
TCRp55[b]	IL-2	-
TCRp75	IL-2	
VEGFR	VEGF	-
TNFRp55[b]	TNF-α	-
TNFRp70-75	TNF-α	
IL-6R	IL-6	-
IL-6Rp130[b]	IL-6	Oncostatin M, LIF
GM-CSFR[b]	GMCSF	-
MGSAp50	MGSA/*gro*	IL-8
MGSAp70	MGSA/*gro*	

[a]70 kDa low-affinity receptor; *trk* high-affinity receptors only sporadically expressed.

[b]RT-PCF analysis for specific mRNA (Mattei et al, in preparation).

in the microenvironment. In a transgenic mouse fibrosarcoma model, Kandel et al[187] found bFGF in cells of all stages of progression but, extracellular bFGF was detected only in the most malignant lesions. These lesions also showed the highest degrees of neovascularization, suggesting that tumor-derived bFGF contributes to vascularization in this model.

The activation of the proteolytic enzymes tissue-type plasminogen activator (tPA), urokinase-type plasminogen activator (uPA),[188] and collagenases[189] by bFGF might play a role in determining melanoma progression because increased proteolytic activity would allow invasion of cells into surrounding tissues, including the lymphatic and blood vessels.

The FGF receptor family[190] may play a crucial role in melanoma development. FGFR-1 is expressed as a single 3.5 kb mRNA tran-script in normal melanocytes and melanoma cells.[191] Antisense oligodeoxynucleotides targeted against the translation start site and a splice donor-acceptor site of human FGFR-1 inhibited proliferation of melanocytes and melanoma cells and also caused extensive dendrite formation.[191] These results support the previous finding with the ligand that bFGF is an autocrine growth factor in melanoma.

In addition to bFGF, three other members of the FGF family, the K-*fgf/hst*, *int-2*, KGF genes, are expressed in human melanoma cells.[192,193] In contrast to the bFGF gene, which does not appear to be amplified or grossly rearranged in melanoma,[193] the K-*fgf/hst* and *int-2* genes have shown evidence of amplification in 2 of 21 melanoma specimens examined.[192,193] The biological significance of this amplification remains to be investigated.

Table 20. Constitutive expression of growth factor genes by melanoma cells[a]

Growth factor	Cell line in growth factor-free medium				
	WM983B	WM164	WM239A	WM852	WM35
PDGF-α	+	-	+	+	+
PDGF-β	-	-	-	+	-
TGF-β	+	-	+	+	-
TGF-α	-	+	+	+	+
bFGF	+	+	+	+	+
MGSA	+	-	-	-	-
IL-1α	-	-	-	-	+
IL-1β	+	-	-	+	+
IL-3	-	-	-	-	-
Total	6/9	2/9	4/9	6/9	5/9

[a]From Rodeck et al, 1991.

+ = positive expression of mRNA and/or protein; - = no expression.

Table 21. Roles for melanoma-derived growth factors and cytokines

Autocrine growth factors for melanoma cells	Melanoma-derived angiogenic factors	Melanoma-derived mitogens for fibroblasts	Melanoma-derived chemotactic and motility-stimulating factors	
			Chemotaxis	Motility
bFGF	bFGF	bFGF	IL-8	Autocrine motility factor (AMF)
MGSA/gro	PDGF	PDGF	MGSA	IGF-I[a]
IL-6	TGF-α	TGF-α	MCP-1	Chondroitin sulfate proteoglycan
IL-8	TGF-β	TGF-β	M-CSF	$\alpha_4\beta_1$
	TNF-α		GM-CSF	
	pleiotrophin			

[a]Not produced by melanoma cells, but possibly induced in juxtaposed fibroblasts.

TGF-α

TGF-α belongs to the epidermal growth factor (EGF) family of mitogens.[194] EGF and TGF-α have closely related tertiary structures based on the homologous spacing of cysteine residues that form three intracellular disulfide bonds. TGF-α competes with EGF for binding to the EGF-receptor. Although TGF-α-like proteins of high molecular weight appear to be expressed and/or secreted by various transformed cells, the fully processed, mature form of TGF-α (56 kDa) is a monomeric 50 amino acid protein encoded by an mRNA of approximately 4,800 bases.[195]

TGF-α was one of the first melanoma-derived growth factors to be reported.[196,197] Melanoma cells often produce and secrete large quantities of TGF-α-like factors as compared to other tumor cell lines.[198-200] Low molecular weight[201,202] and high molecular weight[203] species of TGF-α-like activities have been detected in the urine of melanoma patients. Whether melanoma cells also express the cell surface-bound TGF-α is not known. It also remains to be determined whether TGF-α in the urine of melanoma patients is tumor- or host-derived. In this respect, Hudgins et al[203] detected rat EGF but not human EGF or TGF-α in the urine of nude rats xenotransplanted with human lung carcinoma or chondrosarcoma cells. In a recent survey, four of five melanoma cell lines constitutively expressed TGF-α transcripts. This finding is in accord with other reports describing expression of the TGF-α gene in fresh melanoma tissue specimens[204] and in melanoma cell lines.[205] No TGF-α transcripts have been detected in normal melanocyte RNA [U. Rodeck, unpublished] nor do normal melanocytes in vitro produce detectable quantities of TGF-α unless stimulated by UV irradiation.[206] This stimulation appears to be a posttranslational event.[207]

Expression of the EGF/TGF-α receptor in cultured melanoma cells, as determined by the binding of an EGF receptor-specific MAb, correlates with an increased dosage of chromosome 7.[208] In situ, expression of the EGF receptor correlates with tumor progression.[209,210] The EGF receptor is not detected on normal melanocytes and common acquired nevi, is expressed in approximately 20% of dysplastic nevi and RGP primary melanomas, and is highly expressed in VGP primary

---

Table 22. Activation of growth factors and cytokine expression by other factors[a]

		Activation by exogenous			
IL-1	IL-6	IL-8	G-CSF/GM-CSF	MGSA	PDGF
IL-1[b]	IL-1	IL-1	IL-1	IL-1	PDGF
TNF-α	TNF-α	TNF-α	TNF-α	TNF-α	IL-1
IFN-γ				MGSA	MGSA
IL-6					
MGSA					

[a]Studies mostly done using fibroblasts and endothelial cells. (For more details see Herlyn and Malkowicz, 1991).

[b]Activated factor.

(89%) and metastatic melanoma (80%).[210,211] TGF-α and EGF-receptor mRNA transcripts appear to be coordinately expressed within the same lesion.[204] Exogenous EGF moderately stimulates the growth of some melanoma cells,[212,213] suggesting that the receptor is functional. The mitogenic effects of EGF in vitro appear to depend at least in part on culture conditions. Normal melanocytes and melanoma cells at early passages respond to EGF, whereas established melanocyte cultures do not.[214,215]

Although TGF-α and immunoreactive EGF/TGF-α receptor are co-expressed by some melanoma cells, no direct evidence supporting an autocrine role for melanoma-derived TGF-α is available. We have used EGF receptor-reactive MAb 425, which is an EGF/TGF-α antagonist, to demonstrate the autocrine function of TGF-α for carcinoma cells.[216] In defined culture media that do not contain exogenous EGF/TGF-α, MAb 425 has no reproducible inhibitory effect on growth of melanoma cells that coordinately express TGF-α and EGF receptors [U. Rodeck, unpublished]. This finding is in agreement with an earlier report that described lack of growth inhibition of melanoma cells by an EGF-antagonistic MAb to the intact EGF receptor.[217] Based on these findings, we conclude that secreted, melanoma-derived TGF-α is not essential for melanoma cell proliferation in vitro. However, it may have paracrine angiogenic and mitogenic functions (Table 21).

TGF-β

TGF-β is structurally and functionally distinct from TGF-α. Mature and bioactive TGF-β (25 kDa) consists of two disulfide-bonded subunits of 112 amino acids each [see ref. 218 for review]. Five closely related isoforms have been cloned. Mature TGF-β is the product of complex proteolytic processing of much larger precursor molecules. Pro-TGF-β is a non-covalently-linked complex, consisting of the precursor peptide and the mature TGF-β dimer. Further processing is required to release the biologically active mature TGF-β polypeptide. Bioactive TGF-β binds to high-affinity cell surface receptors

that are as yet poorly characterized. TGF-β exerts pleiotropic effects in tissue development, wound healing, and growth regulation.

Active TGF-β appears to have a negative growth regulatory role in the majority of normal and malignant epithelial cells.[219,220] It also inhibits growth of normal melanocytes[221] and melanoma cells in culture.[222] The majority of melanoma lines in culture express TGF-β1 mRNA constitutively.[223,224] DeLarco et al[225] have shown that TGF-β protein is also secreted by melanoma cells in culture. Melanoma cells also express TGF-β2 and TGF-β3.[226] Interestingly, melanocytes do not express mRNA for TGF-β2 but do express TGF-β1 and β3. TGF-β has a variety of paracrine effects which include the downregulation of proteolytic enzymes through the activation of enzyme inhibitors or the increase of extracellular matrix protein production.[227]

The receptors for TGF-β have not yet been investigated in melanoma cells. Massagué[228] distinguished nine different TGF-β binding proteins; whether any of these are biologically relevant is unclear.

PLATELET-DERIVED GROWTH FACTOR (PDGF)

Human PDGF is a dimeric molecule (28-31 kDa) consisting of PDGF-A and/or PDGF-B subunits which are encoded by different genes [see ref. 229 for review]. Both homodimers (PDGF-AA and PDGF-BB), as well as the heterodimer, PDGF-AB, are biologically active and bind with different affinities to the PDGF-α and -β receptors, except that PDGF-AA homodimers do not bind to the PDGF-β receptor. The v-*sis* oncogene of simian sarcoma virus encodes a protein that is homologous to the PDGF-B chain,[230,231] binds to the PDGF receptors,[232] and has been shown to act in an autocrine fashion in simian sarcoma virus-transformed cells.[233]

The expression of either one or both PDGF isoforms and secretion of a mitogen, which appears to be homodimeric PDGF-A, has been observed in human melanoma cells derived from one primary and two metastatic lesions of the same patient, but not in normal melanocytes in culture.[234] Subsequent studies demonstrated PDGF-A mRNA expression in

$3/6^{235}$ or $6/16^{236}$ melanoma cell lines. These results indicate expression of PDGF-A by about 50% of cultured melanoma lines, whereas expression of PDGF-B appears to be less frequent. Most melanoma cells do not express detectable PDGF receptors at the cell surface in ligand binding assays (B. Westermark, personal communication). However, radiolabeled exogenous PDGF appears to be translocated to the nucleus of melanoma cells,[237,238] suggesting a low-level expression of receptor proteins. Harsh et al[239] reported the expression of PDGF-receptor genes in 3/8 melanoma cell lines tested. We have observed low-level expression of the PDGF-β-receptor mRNA in one of four melanoma lines tested. That cell line also expressed PDGF-A and PDGF-B transcripts. It is not known whether the lack of PDGF-receptor expression on the membrane is due to downregulation by endogenous ligand. Exogenous PDGF is not mitogenic for melanoma cells in short-term [³H]thymidine incorporation assays or in long-term cell proliferation assays. Neutralizing polyclonal antisera, specific for PDGF, do not inhibit proliferation of PDGF-producing melanoma cells. Although it cannot be excluded at present that endogenous PDGF stimulates PDGF receptors at an intracellular location inaccessible to blocking antibodies,[240] no evidence for an autocrine role of this factor is currently available.

PDGF appears to have paracrine function in melanoma.[241] When melanoma cells that do not produce any of the PDGFs are transfected with PDGF-B, they proliferate more rapidly in vivo. Transfected cells induce tumors with an abundance of blood vessels in the connective tissue septa and within the tumor cell stroma. These tumors, in contrast to those induced by the parental cells, have no central necrosis. The connective tissue network that is generated in response to PDGF-BB homodimers may form a solid support for newly formed blood vessels and thereby facilitate the formation of a functional vascular system in the tumor.

PLEIOTROPHIN

Pleiotrophin (heparin-binding growth associated molecule [HB-GAM], heparin-

binding neurotrophic factor [HBNF]) is a developmentally regulated, neurotrophic factor secreted by melanoma cells.[242] It is an 18 kDa protein that has functional similarities with bFGF.[243-246] It is also secreted by breast carcinoma cells[247] and its activity can be inhibited by heparin analogs.[247] Pleiotrophin is highly angiogenic. Inhibitors of pleiotrophin such as pentosanpolysulfate can inhibit metastasis formation by limiting tumor growth at the metastatic sites. Melanoma cells do not appear to express the receptor for pleiotrophin (A. Wellstein, personal communication). Therefore, melanoma-derived pleiotrophin might play a major paracrine role in angiogenesis.

MGSA/GRO AND IL-8

MGSA (melanocyte growth stimulatory activity) was first isolated from conditioned media of the melanoma cell line Hs0294T and is identical to the *gro* gene product,[248] which belongs to the family of monocyte inflammatory proteins (MIP-2).[249] The bioactivity of MGSA is found primarily in polypeptides ranging from 14 to 28 kDa.[250] The fully processed mature form of the MGSA appears to be at most 73 amino acids long. The deduced amino acid sequence of MGSA reveals extensive similarities to the precursor of b-thromboglobulin and connective tissue-activating protein, heparin-binding platelet factor-4, the interferon-γ inducible gene γIP-10, and IL-8/NAP-3.[251,25] In addition to its mitogenic activity, MGSA appears to be a mediator of chemotaxis and inflammation, with strong neurotrophic properties (Table 21).

MGSA binds to the surface of, and is a mitogen for, Hs0294T melanoma cells which produce this factor.[253,254] An MAb that binds to MGSA inhibited growth of Hs0294T cells, indicating that MGSA has an autocrine function in this cell line,[255] although effects of the MAb on the proliferation of other melanoma cell lines have not been reported. Northern blot analysis of total RNA preparations from Hs0294T cells grown in serum-free media revealed low-level or absent expression of MGSA.[256] In another study, none of five melanoma cell lines expressed MGSA transcript constitutively when grown in culture medium free of exogenous growth factors

(Table 20).[257] However, Chevenix-Trent et al[258] have detected MGSA transcripts not only in the majority of melanoma cells tested, but also in normal melanocytes. These discrepancies might be explained by different culture conditions, since MGSA production is inducible when exogenous mitogens such as PDGF and MGSA are added to the culture medium.[256] The receptor for MGSA is a dimer with 50-58 kDa and 70-78 kDa subunits.[259,260] On Hs0294T melanoma cells, Horuk et al[261] detected a unique MGSA receptor which bound only MGSA and not IL-8. On U937 leukemia cells, on the other hand, MGSA and IL-8 competed for the same receptor.

IL-8 is secreted by most if not all melanoma cells in culture (M. Colombo, D. Guerry IV, personal communications). It is a 8 kDa protein that is chemotactic for neutrophils, T cells, and basophils. Neutrophils are the apparent natural source for IL-8.[262] It also induces migration of melanoma cells (Table 21).[263] IL-8 is produced by many different tumors of neuoectodermal origin.[264] It stimulates intracellular calcium transiently and promotes keratinocyte proliferation, apparently in an autocrine fashion.[265] IL-8 may act as an autocrine growth factor for melanoma cells (D. Schadendorf, personal communication). The protein γIP-10, which is related to MGSA and IL-8, is also produced by melanoma cells.[266] IL-8, MGSA, or platelet factor 4 can decrease collagen synthesis by human fibroblasts.[267]

IL-1 AND IL-6

IL-1 was originally purified from monocytes;[268] however, it is produced in a variety of cell types as developmentally diverse as lymphoid cells, endothelial cells, fibroblasts, and keratinocytes [see ref. 269 for review]. Two distinct forms IL-1α and IL-1β, encoded by separate genes have been identified. These isoforms share the same molecular mass (18 kDa) and a common cell surface receptor.

Both IL-1α and IL-1β are present in conditioned media of monocytes and are strong inhibitors of the proliferation of A375 human melanoma cells.[270,271] In another study, IL-1β significantly inhibited [³H]thymidine incor-

poration of 3/9 melanoma cell lines.[272] By contrast, coinjection of IL-1 and a variant of A375 melanoma cells enhanced the formation of metastatic foci in the lungs of recipient athymic mice.[273]

Cultured human melanoma cells are not only the target, but also a source of both isoforms of bioactive IL-1.[274-276] IL-1 was produced by 16 of 27 metastatic melanoma cell lines tested. Secreted and cell-associated forms have been identified. Cloning of IL-1α and IL-1β from a melanoma library revealed sequence identity to the monocyte-derived forms.[278] It is unclear at present whether melanoma-derived IL-1 modulates growth of the producing cells. However, it appears possible that IL-1 in vivo acts primarily in a paracrine fashion (Table 22). Rice and Bevilacqua[277] have shown that IL-1 induces an adhesion molecule on the surface of cultured endothelial cells (INCAM-110/V-CAM-1) which mediates the attachment of melanoma cells to activated endothelium. Thus, cell-associated melanoma-derived IL-1 may facilitate metastatic spread by enhancing tumor cell/endothelial cell adhesion. In light of the ability of IL-1 to activate the expression of a number of different cytokines such as TNF-α, interferon-γ, and IL-6 (Table 22), most of which can be produced by melanoma cells (Table 18), it may be that IL-1 plays an important role in tumorigenesis. Melanoma-derived IL-1 can upregulate ICAM-1 and ELAM-1 expression on endothelial cells[279] in addition to V-CAM-1, which might further increase metastatic potential.

The significance of IL-6 production by melanoma cells or the role of IL-6 as a paracrine stimulator has recently been investigated by Kerbel and co-workers.[280-282] IL-6 shows a growth inhibitory function on melanoma cells.[283] However, primary melanoma cells may act differently than metastatic cells. Whereas RGP and VGP primary melanoma cells were inhibited by fibroblast-derived IL-6, metastatic cells were not.[280,282] Since IL-6 is produced by metastatic melanoma cells,[281,284] it is conceivable that IL-6 acts as an autocrine factor in melanoma.[282] gp 130,[285-287] the coreceptor for IL-6 and other members of this family, i.e., oncostatin M and LIF (leukemia inhibitory factor), is expressed by melanoma cells.[288] Whether oncostatin M and LIF play a role in melanoma biology is currently under investigation in different laboratories. LIF mRNA is found in most melanomas,[288] and LIF-producing melanoma cells induce cachexis when injected into nude mice.[289] Oncostatin M, but not LIF, is inhibitory for primary melanoma cells. [R. Kerbel, personal communication.]

IGF-I AND SCATTER FACTOR

IGF-I and insulin are potent exogenous growth factors for cultured melanoma cells.[290] Melanoma cells express the IGF-I receptor, and the mitogenic effects of both insulin and IGF-I are significantly inhibited by a MAb to the IGF-I receptor that inhibits binding of these ligands. Of a panel of six human melanoma cell lines tested, none produced IGF-I or IGF-II proteins (R. Furlanetto, personal communication), nor did any express detectable mRNA transcripts for these two factors.[291] IGF-I is a motility factor for melanoma cells (Table 21).[292,293] Since IGF-I can be produced by fibroblasts, it is conceivable that it is an important paracrine stimulator of melanoma cells.

Scatter factor (hepatocyte growth factor) is another fibroblast-derived growth factor that stimulates cell motility.[294] The receptor for scatter factor, *met*, is found in many different malignant tumors,[295] including melanomas.[296] On normal melanocytes, scatter factor acts synergistically with bFGF. Both factors may contribute to melanoma development: bFGF by growth promotion and angiogenesis, and scatter factor by dispersion of cells allowing them to separate from the primary nodule.

OTHER FACTORS

Melanocyte-stimulating hormone (MSH) and the related melanotropins are pituitary-derived peptides that have widely divergent effects on the growth of non-human melanocytes [see ref. 297 for review]. Human melanoma cell lines and melanoma tumors express melanotropin receptors.[298-300] Recently, it was reported that metastatic melanoma lesions simultaneously express MSH receptors and contain immunoreactive α-MSH protein.[301] These findings suggest a potential autocrine role for this factor. However, Ellem and Kay[302] reported that exogenous α-MSH did not affect proliferation of human melanoma cells MM96. MSH is involved in the induction of pigmentation in melanocytes.[303,304] It remains to be determined whether this hormone has additional growth regulatory functions. Several MSH receptors have been cloned and preliminarily characterized.[305,306] Of the potentially eight different receptors, three have been found on melanoma cells (H. Eberle, personal communication). MSH-receptors define a subfamily of receptors coupled to guanine nucleotide-binding proteins that activate adenylcyclase. MSH receptors are overexpressed in melanoma cells[305] but they can also be found in a variety of tissues.

Two endothelial cell mitogens, platelet-derived endothelial cell growth factor (ECGF)[307] and vascular endothelial cell growth factor (VEGF), or vascular permeability factor,[308] play potential roles in melanoma tumorigenesis. The receptor for VEGF is expressed by melanoma cells but not melanocytes.[309] ECGF mRNA is expressed by melanoma cells when tested by RT-RCR (M. Colombo, unpublished).

Several melanoma-derived growth inhibitory factors have been documented to inhibit growth of some melanoma cells when added exogenously to cultures. Growth inhibitory effects of exogenous bioactive TGF-β and IL-1 have been described in Chapters 5. A melanoma-inhibitory activity (MIA) was described[310-312] that was purified from the conditioned medium of a human metastatic melanoma cell line (HTZ 19-dM) and, after purification, inhibited proliferation of the producing cells. This factor (8 kDa) is apparently unrelated to TGF-β and IL-1, but the structure of the protein and the coding sequence have not been determined. Other inhibitory factors of melanoma cells are TNF-α,[313] IL-6, oncostatin M, interferon-α, interferon-β,[314] and Mullerian inhibitory substance[315] (Table 23).

Of all the growth factors, cytokines, and receptors studied to date, only few show discordant expression, i.e., absence of either ligand or receptor (Table 24). This infrequence of discordance is quite remarkable and suggests that melanoma cells may have multiple autocrine loops for a variety of functions. Table 24 lists also those growth factors and cytokines that have the respective receptor concomitantly expressed. Studying the regulation of the expression of these genes will be a major challenge for researchers seeking to understand the biology of melanomas.

PROTEIN TYROSINE KINASES AND PROTEIN KINASES

Protein tyrosine kinases play a key role in the control of cell proliferation and differentiation. These proteins are either transmembrane receptors for polypeptide growth factors or cytoplasmic kinases often implicated in signal transduction from other receptors.

They include many oncogene products, several of which are receptors.[316,317] A role for protein tyrosine kinases in melanoma is supported by the expression of various oncogenes and growth factor receptors. Bennett and collaborators recently conducted an investigation of the expression of tyrosine protein kinases in melanoma.[318] Initial screening was done by RT-PCR followed by Northern blotting (Table 25). Easty et al[318] found kinases of several families, most notably of the EPH and FGF receptor families. D. Bennett, R. Spritz, and N. Lassam have independently also found melanocyte-specific kinases (personal communications). Four patterns of expression are found: 1) expression in melanomas but not melanocytes; 2) expression at similar levels in normal melanocytes and melanomas; 3) expression in melanocytes but not melanomas; and 4) expression in both melanocytes and melanomas but overexpression in melanomas. The contribution

Table 23. Factors that are inhibitory for melanoma cells

Factor	Inhibition[a]	Expresison by melanoma[b]
TGF-β[c]	++++	+
IL-6[d]	++[c]	+
Oncostatin M[d]	+++[c]	?
Mullerian inhibitory substance	++	?
TNF-α	++	+
IL-1	+	+
Interferon-β	+++	+
Interferon-α	++	-
Interferon-γ	++	-
MIA	+++	+

[a]+ → ++++ relative degree of inhibition.
[b]As tested by mRNA or protein assays.
[c]Some metastatic cells may be resistant.
[d]Primary melanomas only.

of individual protein tyrosine kinase to melanoma development and progression needs further clarification.

The important roles for protein kinases in melanoma is highlighted by the striking effect of the protein kinase C (PK-C) activator TPA as a growth stimulator for melanocytes and growth inhibitor for melanoma cells (see Chapter 4). Becker et al[319] found PK-Cα expression in primary and metastatic melanomas but not in melanocytes, whereas Meyskens and coworkers[320] found three isotypes, α, β, and ε, constitutively expressed in melanocytes and α and ε expressed in melanomas. Other investigators have also found PK-Cα and ε in melanocytes.[321] TPA leads to a high level of phosphorylation of a major substrate, the myristoylated alanine-rich C kinase substrate protein (MARCKS). In melanoma, TPA induces transient cell arrest and inhibits the phosphorylation of p34cdc^2.[322] Differentiation of murine melanoma cells by retinoic acid is preceded by a large increase of PK-Cα mRNA and protein.[323] PK-Cα-transfected melanoma cells show reduced tumorigenicity. These preliminary efforts point to a crucial role for PKs in melanoma growth and differentiation, but the mechanisms are still unclear.

CATION-BINDING PROTEINS

Melanoma cells overexpress a large number of calcium-binding proteins (Table 26).

The calcium-binding S-100 protein is a highly acidic cytoplasmic protein with a molecular mass of 21 kDa when isolated from bovine brain extracts.[324] It is composed of two peptide chains which associate as dimers.[325] The S-100 protein is part of a family of calcium-binding proteins, which VanEldik[326] called calcium-modulating proteins and which include calmodulin. Although S-100 protein is highly characteristic of neural crest-derived tumors, including melanoma,[327] it is also detected in other normal and malignant tissues.[328] Antibodies to S-100 are widely used for the immunohistological diagnosis of non-pigmented melanomas.[329] S-100b protein binds to tumor suppressor p53 in a calcium-dependent manner, and the gene localizes to a chromosomal region on the tip of 219 that was recently linked to melanoma susceptibility in several Australian pedigrees.

Calmodulin is a small (17 kDa) monomeric protein with four Ca^{++} binding domains and is present in virtually all eukaryotes. Calmodulin modulates the activity of

---

Table 24. Discordant and concomitant expression of cytokines and growth factors with their receptors by melanoma cells

Ligand positive/ Receptor negative	Ligand negative/ Receptor positive	Ligand positive/ Receptor positive
PDGF A and B	IGF-I	bFGF
pleiotrophin[a]	Scatter factor	TGF-α
	Interferon-α and -γ	TGF-β
	IL-2	*steel*
	IL-3	
	IL-4	IL-1
		IL-6
		IL-7
		IL-8
		MGSA
		TNFα
		GM-CSF

[a]Receptor not yet identified but apparently absent on melanoma cells. (A. Wellstein, personal communication).

several key enzymes and other factors in growth regulation. Three genes, CAM I, II, and III, encode a single protein. mRNA analysis of melanocytes and metastatic melanomas revealed qualitative and quantitative differences in expression.[329] Addition of serum enhanced CAM I and II expression in melanocytes and TPA strongly enhanced CAM I expression.[329]

High-level expression of the calcium-binding calcyclin was detected on metastatic melanoma cells when compared to primary cells,[330] and calnexin (calreticulin) was similarly overexpressed in metastatic melanoma cells (K. Jimbow, personal communication). The functional role of overexpressed calcium-binding proteins in melanoma cells remains unclear.

The p97 molecule is very immunogenic in mice and many MAbs have been produced in different laboratories. Brown, Hellström and their associates have studied the tissue distribution of p97 extensively.[331-333] In culture,

Table 25. Protein tyrosine kinases expressed by melanoma cells[a]

Family	Kinase receptors
EPH	TYRO-6
	ECK
	TYRO-4
FGF-R	FGF-R4/TKF
	TYRO-9
INS-R	TGF-I-R
TYRO-3	TYRO-3
NGF-R	TYRO-10
?	JTK
	Cytoplasmic
CSK	CSK/TYRO-13
FES	FES

[a]From Easty et al, submitted.

Table 26. Cation-binding proteins expressed by melanoma cells

Antigen	Cation
S-100a	Calcium
S-100b	Calcium
Calnexin (Calreticulin)	Calcium
Calmodulin	Calcium
Calcyclin	Calcium
p97 melanotransferrin	Iron, zinc
Tyrosinase	Copper

this protein is highly expressed by almost all melanoma cells as well as by a few carcinomas. In situ, most melanomas bind MAbs to p97. In fetal tissues, p97 is found mostly in the colonic mucosa and in adult tissues on sweat gland cells.

There are at least five different antigenic determinants on p97.[334] The protein is a monomeric sialoglycoprotein with intrachain disulfide bonds. N-terminal amino acid sequencing revealed homology in 7 of 12 residues with transferrin and lactotransferrin[335] and since purified p97 can bind iron, it has a functional relationship to transferrin.

Purified and cloned p97 mRNA encodes a 738-residue precursor, and the mature p97 molecule comprises extracellular domains of 342 and 352 residues and a C-terminal 25-residue stretch of predominantly uncharged and hydrophobic amino acids, which may act as a membrane anchor.[336,337] Each extracellular domain contains 14 cysteine residues, which form 7 intradomain disulfide bridges, and possibly one or two glycosylation sites. The conservation of disulfide bridges and amino acids thought to compose the iron binding pockets suggest that p97 is also related to transferrin in tertiary structure and function. This has led Rose et al[336] to suggest the name "melanotransferrin" for p97. Based on a molecular model of p97,[338] it appears that p97 also has zinc-binding properties.

Histochemical determinations of copper, zinc, and iron revealed the increased presence of copper and iron in melanomas when compared to nevi.[339] Studies on cultured cells also showed that copper and iron are important components of medium W487 for melanocytes.[340] Copper may be bound by tyrosinase and ceruloplasmin, whereas iron is bound by transferrin and melanotransferrin.

PROTEOLYTIC ENZYMES AND THEIR INHIBITORS

Melanoma cells are very active secretors of proteases that are thought to be involved in invasion and metastasis [see ref. 341 for recent review]. As summarized in Table 27, at least five groups of proteases can be found in the culture supernatant of melanoma cells. These include the serine protease tissue-type and uroki-nase-type plasminogen activator,[342-345] metalloproteinases collagenases type IV (72 and 92 kDa),[346,347] interstitial collagenase and stromelysin, heparanase, cathepsins,[348] and tissue factor.[349] Of the type IV collagenases, the 72 kDa form is predominantly found. Expression of enzymes is heterogenous and regulated by various growth factors and cytokines, most notably bFGF, IL-1, and TGF-β.[341] The proteases are secreted as inactive precursors that require activation by other proteases.

Expression of proteolytic enzymes is also regulated by specific inhibitors. As summarized in Table 28, melanoma cells express inhibitors for collagenase type IV and plasminogen activators including TIMPs (tissue inhibitor for metalloproteinases) and PAIs (plasminogen activator inhibitors). α_2-Macroglobulin is a protease inhibitor on melanoma cells[350] that binds several growth factors, most notably TGF-β. The dynamics of activation of proteolytic enzymes during invasion and metastasis has recently been reviewed.[341] However, further studies are needed to determine the melanoma specificity of such interactions. The expression of serine and metalloproteinases appears to be a reliable marker for progression but more detailed analyses are needed.

Cell surface proteases form a separate class of proteases (Table 29). They have a less restricted specificity and their function is little understood. Aminopeptidase N appears to be involved in invasion by digesting nidogen/entactin.[351] Neither the role of leucine aminopeptidase in differentiated melanoma cells[352] nor the functions of neutral endopeptidase and of cell surface gelatinase are clear.

MELANOCYTE LINEAGE MARKERS

Table 30 summarizes the melanocyte lineage markers that are potentially important for melanocyte/melanoma biology and the immunological identification of melanocytic cells. These structures may be detected by molecular techniques, histochemistry or immunohistology. Several markers, such as S-100 and the 100/7 kDa HMB-45 antigen are not melanocyte lineage-specific, but can be used in combination with other markers for the identification of melanoma cells.

Table 27. Proteases secreted by melanoma cells

Enzyme	Substrate	Regulation[a]
Plasminogen activators urokinase type (uPA) tissue type (tPA)	Plasminogen	bFGF↑ IL-1↑ TGF-β↓
Collagenases 72 kDa (gelatinase A) 92 kDa (gelatinase B)	 Collagen types IV, V, VI and others Collagen types IV, V, VI and others	 bFGF↑ IL-1↑ TGF-β↓
Interstitial collagenase	Collagen types I, II, III	
Stromelysin	Proteoglycan, laminin, fibrinogen, collagens	IL-1↑ IL-6↑ TGF-β↓
Heparanase	Heparan sulfate proteoglycan	
Cathepsins D and H	Fibrinogen, fibronectin	TGF-β↓
Tissue factor	Factor VIIa for coagulation cascade	

[a]Modulation by exogenous factors (most studies done in fibroblasts and endothelial cells).

↓, Downregulator; ↑, Upregulator.

Table 28. Protease inhibitors expressed by melanoma cells

Inhibitor	Substrate	Regulation
TIMP-1 (28 kDa) glycosylated	92 K gelatinase	TGF-β↑
TIMP-2 (21 kDa) nonglycosylated	72 K gelatinase	TGF-β↓
PAI-1	Plasminogen activators	TGF-β↑
PAI-2		
α2-macroglobulin		Binds TGF-β

Melanin production is the main function of normal melanocytes located in the epidermis. The numbers of melanosomes (the specific secretory granules of melanocytes) and the level of melanin production increase with melanocyte maturation. Melanocytes cultured in TPA-containing medium retain their mature phenotype. Melanoma cells present all grades of pigmentation from a seemingly normal pigment content to an amelanotic appearance. Consequently, much attention has focused on functional and structural changes of melanogenesis during melanocytic tumor progression.

One of the key enzymes for melanin synthesis is tyrosinase. Tyrosinase hydroxylates tyrosine and oxidizes dopa 5,6-dihydroxyindole. Using a MAb against human tyrosinase, McEwan et al[353] found no significant correlation between tyrosinase levels and melanoma tumor progression; even amelanotic melanomas had detectable tyrosinase activity.

Melanoma cells synthesize melanosomes that are disarranged in their melanosomal matrix protein composition.[354] Several MAbs have been generated against structural proteins of melanosomes in melanoma cells. Among these MAbs, HMSA 1, HMSA 2, HMSA 3, HMSA 4, and HMSA 6 are reactive only with melanoma cells and not with normal melanocytes.[355-358]

Another protein of importance for melanin production is gp 75 (HMSA 5, TRP-1), which demonstrates homology with the mouse b (brown) gene[359] and has catalase activity (catalase B).[360] Expression of this protein correlates with pigmentation of melanocytes and melanoma cells in culture.[361] The brown locus (CAS 2) is on human chromosome 9p23,[362,363] a region which is frequently altered in melanoma. gp 75 is synthesized as a 55 kDa polypeptide, glycosylated by addition and processing of five or more Asn-linked carbohydrate chains through the *cis* and Golgi, and transported to melanosomes as a mature 75 kDa form.[364] Orlow et al[365] found an overlap in the distribution of gp 75 (TRP-1) and lysosome-associated membrane protein-1 (LAMP-1). Another melanoma marker, ME491 (neuroglandular antigen, CD63; See Chapter 5), is also a lysosomal membrane protein. However, the function and significance of these markers are not yet clear. Kwon identified the melanocyte-specific gene Pmel17, coding for the silver coat locus on mouse chromosome 10 and human chromosome 12.[366]

MISCELLANEOUS MELANOMA-ASSOCIATED ANTIGENS

The spectrum of melanoma-associated antigens can be extended to those that have membrane transport functions (multidrug resistance gene-1, MDR-1) and those involved in cell growth (Ki67 and 4F2) or transcription (Oct-M2) (Table 31). Two major melanoma-associated antigens, chondroitin sulfate proteoglycan and the neuroglandular antigen ME491, have functions not yet clearly defined.

Table 29. Cell surface proteases expressed by melanoma cells

Protease	Alternative code
Neutral endopeptidase	Calla, 95-100 kDa, CD10
Aminopeptidase N 143 kDa	CD13
Leucine aminopeptidase	LAP
Gelatinase	Invadopodia-associated gelatinase, 170 kDa

The ME491 antigen[367,368] is localized on the lysosomal membrane and the cell surface and might be a transport protein. It was one of the first tumor antigens cloned.[369] It is a highly glycosylated protein with a core of 20 kDa.[370-377] Tissue expression, intracellular location and structure and synthesis have recently been characterized. The protein sequence shows considerable homology with CD9,[378] CD37,[379] CD53,[380] TAPA-1,[381] CO-29,[382] R2,[383] and the Schistosomal membrane protein Sm23.[384] Surprisingly, all antibodies produced in different laboratories to the ME491 antigen compete with each other for binding, probably to the same determinant.[367]

Chondroitin sulfate proteoglycan, also termed high molecular weight melanoma-associated antigen (HMWMAA) might be involved in cell-cell contact, cell-substrate adhesion, or motility. It is a major mela-noma-associated antigen that is highly immunogenic in mice when animals are injected with melanoma cells, nevus cells, or glioma cells.[368] Due to the large molecular mass of the protein core (260 kDa), chondroitin sulfate proteoglycan might also act as a binding protein for growth regulators such as growth factors or proteolytic enzymes. Most melanoma cells express between 100,000 and 6,000,000 binding sites.[385-387] The chondroitin sulfate proteoglycan is expressed on the melanoma cell surface as microspikes which are present as 1-2 μm structures on the upper cell surface and as structures of up to 20 μm at the cell periphery.[388] Peripheral chondroitin sulfate proteoglycan microspikes are involved in the initial interactions between adjacent cells and they form complex footpads that make contact with the substratum. Expression of chondroitin sulfate proteoglycan was induced

Table 30. Melanocyte lineage markers[a]

Antigen	MAb
Tyrosinase (albino [c] locus)	—
gp 75 (brown [b] locus; TRP-1)	TA99
	2G10
	HMSA-5
TRP-2 (Slaty locus)	—
HMSA-1 (20 kDa core protein)	HMSA-1
HMSA-6 (41/22/17/11 kDa)	HMSA-6
100/7 kDa[b]	HMB-45
	NKI-beteb
100/10 kDa[b]	HMB-50
Dopa-oxidase	—
Melanin	—
S-100[b]	Many
Pmel17 (silver coat locus)	—

[a]List was compiled at the Melanoma Antigen Conference, November 1992, Lausanne, Switzerland.

[b]In combination with other markers.

in human tumor-mouse hybrid cells when cells were cultured on extracellular matrix instead of on plastic,[389] indicating that cell-matrix interactions provide control signals for expression. The antigen is abundantly present in adhesion plaques that are deposited along cell membranes. MAbs to chondroitin sulfate proteoglycan do not significantly affect adhesion of melanoma cells but block chemotactic and chemokinetic motility of the cells[390] and reduce their colony formation in soft agar.[388] Recently, McCarthy and co-workers[391] have provided the first evidence that chondroitin sulfate proteoglycan on melanoma cells is a cell-substrate adhesion receptor that cooperates with the $\alpha_4\beta_1$ adhesion receptor in binding to a heparin-binding domain of fibronectin.

Several distinct epitopes have been detected on chondroitin sulfate proteoglycan with different MAbs defining two,[388,392,393] three,[836,387] and five[390] determinants. Antigenic determinants are located either on the core glycoprotein or on the > 400 kDa chondroitin sulfate proteoglycan,[394,395] with the heterogeneity due largely to the glycosylation of the molecule.[387] [^{3}H]leucine labeling of melanoma cells and digestion of the lysate with chondroitinase ABC showed only the 250 kDa component, whereas lysates of melanoma cells labeled with $^{35}SO_4$-2 revealed only a component of > 400 kDa. The identity of O-linked glycosaminoglycans associated with the chondroitin sulfate proteoglycan was established by alkaline borohydride treatment of $^{35}SO_4$-2-labeled immunoprecipitates and subsequent cellulose acetate electrophoresis. The MAb 9.2.27 recognizes several N-linked glycosylated components at 210 and 220 kDa which may be either degradative components of the core structure or early glycosylated precursors of the 260-kDa core protein.[395] The glycosaminoglycan chains released by alkaline borohydrate treatment of the proteoglycan were approximately 60 kDa. Based on these studies, it was estimated that the core protein has three attached chondroitin sulfate chains.[388]

Table 31. Miscellaneous melanoma-associated antigens involved in transport, cell activation, or ligand binding.

Protein	Function
p170 (MDR-1)	Membrane pump
4F2	Cell activation and transport
Ki67	Cell activation
ME491 (CD63)	Lysosomal transport protein or enzyme?
Chondroitin sulfate proteoglycan	Cell-substrate adhesion
	Cell-cell contact
	Motility
	Ligand binding?
Oct-M2	Transcription?
MAGE I-III	Unknown

The role of Oct-M1 and Oct-M2 is unclear and may be in transcription. These octamers are DNA binding proteins expressed by melanoma cells[396] that are commonly occurring elements of a number of gene promoter and enhancer sequences, and they act as recognition sites for various proteins known as Oct-factors.[397-399]

MAGE I-III peptides have been defined by T lymphocytes.[400] Their functions are unknown.

References

1. Herlyn M, Clark WH Jr, Rodeck U, Mancianit ML, Jambrosic J and Koprowski H: Biology of disease. Biology of tumor progression in human melanocytes. Lab Invest 1987; 56:461-474.

2. Herlyn M and Koprowski H: Melanoma antigens: immunological and biological characterization and clinical significance. Ann Rev Immunol 1988; 6:283-308.

3. Kath R, Rodeck U, Menssen HD, Mancianti M-L, Linnenbach AJ, Elder DE and Herlyn M: Tumor progression in the human melanocytic system. Anticancer Res 1989; 9:865-872.

4. Herlyn M: Human melanoma: Development and progression. Cancer Metastasis Rev 1990; 9:101-112.

5. Herlyn M, Menrad A and Koprowski H: Structure, function, and clinical significance of human tumor antigens. J Natl Cancer Inst 1990; 82:1883-1889.

6. Houghton AN, Herlyn M and Ferrone S: Melanoma antigens. In: Balch C, Houghton A, Milton G and Sober A, eds. Cutaneous melanoma. Philadelphia: J.B. Lippinccott Company, 1992; pp 130-143.

7. Herlyn M, Malkowicz SB: Regulatory pathways in tumor growth and invasion. Lab Invest 1991; 65:262-271.

8. Herlyn M, Rodeck U, Mancianti ML, Cardillo FM, Lang A, Ross AH, Jambrosic J and Koprowski H: Expression of melanoma-associated antigens in rapidly dividing human melanocytes in culture. Cancer Res 1987; 47:3057-3061.

9. Herlyn M, Menrad A. Koprowski H. Structure, function, and clinical significance of human tumor antigens. J Natl Cancer Inst 1990; 82:1883-1889.

10. Hynes RO. Integrins: Versatility, modulation, and signaling in cell adhesion. Cell 1992; 69:11-25.

11. Albelda SM, Buck CA. Integrins and other cell adhesion molecules. FASEB J 1990; 4:2868-2880.

12. Albelda SM, Mette SA, Elder DE, Stewart RM, Damjanovich L, Herlyn M, Buck CA. Integrin distribution in malignant melanoma: Association of the β_3 subunit with tumor progression. Cancer Res 1990; 50:6757-6764.

13. Kramer RH, McDonald KA, Vu MP. Human melanoma cells express a novel integrin receptor for laminin. J Biol Chem 1989; 264:15642-15649.

14. Cheresh DA, Spiro RC. Biosynthetic and functional properties of an Arg-Gly-Asp-directed receptor involved in human melanoma cell attachment to vitronectin, fibrinogen, and von Willebrand factor. J Biol Chem 1987; 262:17703-17711.

15. Klein CE, Steinmayer T, Kaufmann D, Weber L, Brocker EB. Identification of a melanoma progression antigen as integrin VLA-2. J Invest Dermatol 1991; 96:281-284.

16. van Muijen GN, Jansen KF, Cornelissen IM, Smeets DF, Beck JL, Ruiter DJ. Establishment and characterization of a human melanoma cell line (MV3) which is highly metastatic in nude mice. Int J Cancer 1991; 48:85-91.

17. Rice GE, Bevilacqua M. An inducible endothelial cell surface glycoprotein mediates melanoma adhesion. Science 1989; 246:1303-1306.

18. Felding-Habermann B, Ruggeri ZM, Cheresh DA. Distinct biological consequences of integrin $\alpha_v\beta_3$-mediated melanoma cell adhesion to fibrinogen and its plasmic fragments. J Biol Chem 1992; 267:5070-5077.

19. Charo IF, Nannizzi L, Smith JW. Cheresh DA. The vitronectin receptor $\alpha_v\beta_3$ binds fibronectin and acts in concert with a_5b_1 in promoting cellular attachment and spreading on fibronectin. J Cell Biol 1990; 111:2795-2800.

20. Seftor REB, Seftor EA, Gehlsen KR, Stetler-Stevenson WG, Brown PD, Ruoslahti E, Hendrix MJC. Role of the $\alpha_v\beta_3$ integrin in human melanoma cell invasion. Proc Natl Acad Sci USA 1992; 89:1557-1561.

21. Kramer RH, Marks N. Identification of integrin collagen receptors on human melanoma cells. J Biol Chem 1989; 264:4684-4688.

22. Mould AP, Whelden LA, Komoriya A, Wayner EA, Yamada KM, Humphries MJ. Affinity chromatographic isolation of the melanoma adhesion receptor for the IIICS region of fibronectin and its identification as the integrin $\alpha_4\beta_1$. J Biol Chem 1990; 265:4020-4024.

23. Vogel BE, Tarone G, Giancotti FG, Gailit J, Ruoslahti E. A novel fibronectin receptor with an unexpected subunit composition ($\alpha_v\beta_1$). J Biol Chem 1990; 265:5934-5937.

24. Asch AS, Tepler J, Silbiger S, Nachman RL. Cellular attachment to thrombospondin. Cooperative interactions between receptor systems. J Biol Chem 1991; 266:1740-1745.

25. Nip J, Shibata H, Loskutoff DJ, Cheresh DA, Brodt P. Human melanoma cells derived from lymphatic metastases use integrin $\alpha_v\beta_3$ to adhere to lymph node vitronectin. J Clin Invest 1992; 90:1406-1413.

26. Iwamoto Y, Robey FA, Graf J, Sasaki M, Kleinman HK, Yamada Y, Martin GR. YIGSR, a synthetic laminin pentapeptide, inhibits experimental metastasis formation. Science 1987; 238:1132-1134.

27. Liotta LA, Rao CN, Weaver VM. Biochemical interactions of tumor-cells with the basement membrane. Ann Rev Biochem 1986; 55:1037-1057.

28. Graf J, Iwamoto Y, Sasaki M, Martin GR, Kleinman HK, Robey FA, Yamada Y. Identification of an amino acid sequence in laminin mediating cell attachment, chemotaxis, and receptor binding. Cell 1987; 48:989-996.

29. Guo NH, Krutzsch HC, Vogel T, Roberts DD. Interactions of a laminin-binding peptide from a 33-kDa protein related to the 67-kDa laminin receptor with laminin and melanoma cells are heparin-dependent. J Biol Chem 1992; 267:17743-17747.

30. Miyake K, Underhill CB, Lesley J, Kincade PW. Hyaluronate can function as a cell adhesion molecule and CD44 participates in hyaluronate recognition. J Exp Med 1990; 172:69-75.

31. Stamenkovic I, Amiot M, Pesando JM, Seed B. A lymphocyte molecule implicated in lymph node homing as a member of the cartilage link protein family. Cell 1989; 56:1057-1062.

32. Sy MS, Guo YJ, Stamenkovic I. Distinct effects of two CD44 isoform on tumor growth in vivo. J Exp Med 1991; 174:859-866.

33. Günthert U, Hofmann M, Rudy W, Reber S, Zoller M, Haussmann I, Matzku S, Wenzel A, Ponta H, Herrlich P. A new variant of glycoprotein CD44 confers metastatic potential to rat carcinoma cells. Cell 1991; 65:13-24.

34. Arch R, Wirth K, Hormann M, Ponta H, Matzku S, Herrlich P, Zöller M. Participation in normal immune responses of a metastasis-inducing splice variant of CD44. Science 1992; 257:682-685.

35. Goldstin L, Zhou DFH, Picker LJ, Minty CN, Bargatze RF, Ding JF, Butcher EF. A human lymphocyte homing receptor, the Hermes antigen, is related to cartilage proteoglycan core and link proteins. Cell 1989; 56:1063-1072.

36. Thomas L, Etoh T, Stamenkovic I, Mihm MC Jr, Byers HR. Migration of human melanoma cells on hyaluronate is related to CD44 expression. J Invest Dermatol 1993; 100:115-120.

37. Decker M, Chiu ES, Dollbaum C, Moiin A, Hall J, Spendlove R, Longaker MT, Stern R. Hyaluronic acid-stimulating activity in sera from the bovine fetus and from breast cancer patients. Cancer Res 1989; 49:3499-3505.

38. Knudson W, Biswas C, Toole BP. Interactions between human tumor cells and fibroblasts stimulate hyaluronate synthesis. Proc Natl Acad Sci USA 1984; 81:6767-6771.

39. Turley EA, Tretiak M. Glycosaminoglycan production by murine melanoma variants in vivo and in vitro. Cancer Res 1985; 45:5098-5105.

40. Turley EA, Austen L, Vandeligt K, Clary C. Hyaluronan and cell-associated hyaluronan binding protein regulate the locomotion of *ras*-transformed cells. J Cell Biol 1991; 112:1041-1047.

41. Iida J, Skubitz AP, Furcht LT, Wayner EA, McCarthy JB. Coordinate role for cell surface chondroitin sulfate proteoglycan and $\alpha_4\beta_1$ integrin in mediating melanoma cell adhesion to fibronectin. J Cell Biol 1992; 118:431-444.

42. Miller EJ, Herlyn M. The basement membrane in benign and malignant melanocytic lesions. In: Rabes H, Krager S, eds. Contributions to oncology. Switzerland: Basel, 1992; pp 269-282.

43. Stenn KS, Bhawan J. The normal histology of the skin. In: Farmer ER, Hood AF, eds. Pathology of the skin. Norwalk: Appleton and Langer, 1990; pp 3-29.

44. Laurie GW, LeBlond CP, Martin GR. Localization of type-4 collagen, laminin, heparin sulfate proteoglycan, and fibronectin to the basal lamina of basement membranes. J Cell Biol 1982; 95:340-344.

45. Lightner VA, Gumkowski F, Bigner DD, Erickson HP. Tenascin/hexabrachion in human skin: Biochemical identification and localization by light and electron microscopy. J Cell Biol 1989; 108:2483-2493.

46. Fine JD. Antigenic features and structural correlates of basement membranes: Relationship to epidermolysis bullosa. Arch Dermatol 1988; 124:713-717.

47. Fine JD, Horiguchi Y, Jester J, Couchman JR. Detection and partial characterization of a midlamina lucida-hemidesmosome-associated antigen (19-DEJ-1) present within normal skin. J Invest Dermatol 1989; 92:825-830.

48. Zhu XJ, Niimi Y, Bystryn JC. Identification of a 160 kD molecule as a component of the basement membrane zone and as a minor bulluos pemphigoid antigen. J Invest Dermatol 1990; 94:817-821.

49 Wight TN, Raugi GJ, Mumby SM, Bornstein P. Light microscopic immunolocation of thrombospondin in human tissues. J Histochem Cytochem 1985; 33:295-302.

50. Paulsson M, Aumailley M, Deutzmann R, Timpl R, Beck K, Engel J. Laminin-nidogen complex. Extraction with chelating agents and structural characterization. Eur J Biochem 1987; 166:11-19.

51. Kleinman HK, McGarvey ML, Hassell JR, Star VL, Cannon FB, Laurie GW, Martin GR. Basement membrane complexes with biologic activity. Biochemistry 1986; 25:312-318.

52. Lever WF, Schaumberg-Lever G. Melanocyte nevi and malignant melanoma. In: Lever WF, Schaumberg-Lever G, eds. Histopathology of the Skin. Philadelphia: J.B. Lippincott, 1983; pp 681-695.

53. Ranson M, Posen S, Meson RS. Extracellular matrix modulates the function of human melanocytes but not melanoma cells. J Cell Physiol 1991; 136:281-288.

54. Moellmann GE, Kuklinska E, Klaus SN. Observations on the positions of melanocytes with respect to the epidermal basement membrane. J Invest Dermatol 1986; 87:392.

55. Warfvinge K, Agdell J, Andersson L, Andersson A. Attachment and detachment of human epidermal melanocytes. Acta Derm Venereol 1990; 70:189-193.

56. McClenic BK, Mitra RS, Riser BL, Nickoloff BJ, Dixit VM, Varani J. Production and utilization of extracellular matrix components by human melanocytes. Exp Cell Res 1989; 180:314-325.

57. Schmoeckel C, Stolz W, Sakai LY, Burgeson RE, Timpl R, Krieg T. Structure of basement membranes in malignant melanoma and nevocytic nevi. J Invest Dermatol 1989; 92:663-668.

58. Yaar M, Woodley DT, Gilchrest BA. Human nevocellular nevus cells are surrounded by basement membrane components: Immunohistologic studies of human nevus cells and melanocytes in vivo and in vitro. Lab Invest 1988; 58:157-162.

59. Erickson CA. Behavior of neural crest cells on embryonic basal laminae. Dev Biol 1987; 120:38-49.

60. Havenith MG, Van Zandvoort EHM, Cleutjens JP, Bosman FT. Basement membrane deposition in benign and malignant naevo-melanocytic lesions: An immunohistochemical study with antibodies to type IV collagen and laminin. Histopathology 1989; 15:137-146.

61. Beck K, Hunter I, Engel J. Structure and function of laminin: Anatomy of a multidomain glycoprotein. FASEB J 1990; 4:148-160.

62. Kanemoto T, Reich R, Royce L, Greatorex D, Adler SH, Shiraishi N, Martin GR, Yamada Y, Kleinman HK. Identification of an amino acid sequence from the laminin A chain that stimulates metastasis and collagenase IV production. Proc Natl Acad Sci USA 1990; 87:2279-2283.

63. Herlyn M, Graeven U, Speicher D, Sela BA, Bennicelli JL, Kath R, Guerry D IV. Characterization of tenascin secreted by melanoma cells. Cancer Res 1991; 51:4853-4858.

64. Natali PG, Nicotra MR, Bartolazzi A, Mottolese M, Coscia N, Bigotti A, Zardi L. Expression and production of tenascin in benign and malignant lesions of melanocyte lineage. Int J Cancer 1990; 46:586-590.

65. Erickson HP, Bourdon MA. Tenascin: An extracellular matrix protein prominent in specialized embryonic tissues and tumors. Ann Rev Cell Biol 1989; 5:71-92.

66. Chiquet-Ehrismann R, Kalla P, Pearson CA. Participation of tenascin and TGF-β in reciprocal epithelial-mesenchymal interactions of MCF-7 cells and fibroblasts. Cancer Res 1989; 49:4322-4325.

67. Pearson CA, Pearson D, Shibahara S, Hofsteenge J, Chiquet-Ehrismann R. Tenascin: cDNA cloning and induction by TGF-b. EMBO J 1988; 7:2977-2982.

68. Akhurst RJ, Lehnert SA, Faissner A, Duffie E. TGF-β in murine morphogenetic processes: The early embryo and cardiogenesis. Development 1990; 108:645-656.

69. Ruoslahti E, Pierschbacher MD. New perspective in cell adhesion: RGD and integrins. Science 1987; 238:491-497.

70. Soszka T, Knudsen KA, Beviglia L, Rossi C, Poggi A, Niewiarowski S. Inhibition of murine melanoma cell-matrix adhesion and experimental metastasis by albolabrin, an RGD-containing peptide isolated from the venom of Trimeresurus albolaris. Exp Cell Res 1991; 196:6-12.

71. Liotta LA, Rao CN, Weaver VM. Biochemical interactions of tumor-cells with the basement membrane. Ann Rev Biochem 1986; 55:1037-1057.

72. Graf J, Iwamoto Y, Sasaki M, Martin GR, Kleinman HK, Robey FA, Yamada Y. Identification of an amino acid sequence in laminin mediating cell attachment, chemotaxis, and receptor binding. Cell 1987; 49:989-996.

73. Iwamoto Y, Graf J, Sasaki M, Kleinman HK, Greatorex DR, Martin GR, Robey FA, Yamada Y. Synthetic pentapeptide from the B1 chain of laminin promotes B16F10 melanoma cell migration. J Cell Physiol 1988; 134:287-291.

74. Yamamura K, Kibbey MC, Kleinman HK. Melanoma cells selected for adhesion to laminin peptides have different malignant properties. Cancer Res 1993; 53:423-428.

75. Terranova VP. Laminin and fibronectin modulate the metastatic activity of melanoma cells. In: Nathanson L, ed. Basic and clinical aspects of malignant melanoma. Boston: Martinus Nijhoff Publishers, 1987; pp 41-60.

76. McCarthy JB, Skubitz AP, Palm SL, Furcht LT. Metastasis inhibition of different tumor types by purified laminin fragments and a heparin-binding fragment of fibronectin. J Natl Cancer Inst 1988; 80:108-116.

77. Skubitz AP, McCarthy JB, Zhao Q, Yi XY, Furcht LT. Definition of a sequence, RYVVLPR, within laminin peptide F-9 that mediates metastatic fibrosarcoma cell adhesion and spreading. Cancer Res 1990; 50:7612-7622.

78. McCarthy JB, Skubitz AP, Lida J, Mooradian DL, Wilke MS, Furcht LT. Tumor cell adhesive mechanisms and their relationship to metastasis. Semin Cancer Biol 1991; 2:155-167.

79. Skubitz AP, Letourneau PC, Wayner E, Furcht LT. Synthetic peptides from the carboxy-terminal globular domain of the A chain of laminin: Their ability to promote cell adhesion and neurite outgrowth, and interact with heparin, and the beta 1 integrin subunit. J Cell Biol 1991; 115:1137-1148.

80. Mayo KH, Parra-Diaz D, McCarthy JB, Chelberg M. Cell adhesion promoting peptide GVKGDKGNPGWPGAP from the collagen type IV triple helix: cis/trans proline-induced multiple 1H NMR conformations and evidence for a KG/PG multiple turn repeat motif in the all-trans proline state. Biochemistry 1991; 30:8251-8267.

81. Chelberg MK, McCarthy JB, Skubitz AP, Furcht LT, Tsilibary EC. Characterization of a synthetic peptide from type IV collagen that promotes melanoma cell adhesion, spreading, and motility. J Cell Biol 1990; 111:261-270.

82. Guo NH, Krutzsch HC, Negre E, Vogel T, Blake DA, Roberts DD. Heparin- and sulfatide-binding peptides from the type I repeats of human thrombospondin promote melanoma cell adhesion. Proc Natl Acad Sci USA 1992; 89:3040-3044.

83. Öbrink B. C-CAM (cell-CAM 105)—a member of the growing immunoglobulin superfamily of cell adhesion proteins. BioEssays 1991; 13:227-234.

84. Springer TA. Adhesion receptors of the immune system. Nature 1990; 346:425-434.

85. Johnson JP. Cell adhesion molecules of the immunoglobulin supergene family and their role in malignant transformation and progression to metastatic disease. Cancer Metastasis Rev 1991; 10:11-22.

86. Johnson JP. The role of ICAM-1 in tumor development. In: Hogg, N., ed. Chemical Immunology, Karker, Basel. Integrins and ICAM-1 in immune responses. 1991; 50:143-163.

87 Johnson JP, Stade BG, Hoizmann B, Schwable W, Riethmuller G. *De novo* expression of intercellular-adhesion molecule 1 in melanoma correlates with increased risk of metastasis. Proc Natl Acad Sci USA 1989; 86:641-646.

88. Carrel S, Doré J-F, Ruiter DJ, Prade M, Lejeune FJ, Kleeberg UR, Rumke P, Brocker EB. The EORTC melanoma group exchange program: Evaluation of a multicenter monoclonal antibody study. Int J Cancer 1991; 48:836-847.

89. Natali P, Nicotra MR, Cavaliere R, Bigotti A, Romano G, Temponi M, Ferrone S. Differential expression of intercellular adhesion molecule 1 in primary and metastatic melanoma lesions. Cancer Res 1990; 50:1271-1278.

90. Seth R, Raymond FD, Makgoba MW. Circulating ICAM-1 isoforms: Diagnostic prospects for inflammatory and immune disorders. Lancet 1991; 338:83-84.

91. Harning R, Mainolfi E, Bystryn J-C, Henn M, Merluzzi VJ, Rothlein R. Serum levels of circulating intercellular adhesion molecule 1 in human malignant melanoma. Cancer Res 1991; 51:5003-5005.

92. Altomonte M, Colizzi F, Esposito G, Maio M. Circulating intercellular adhesion molecule 1 as a marker of disease progression in cutaneous melanoma. N Engl J Med 1992; 327:959.

93. Mortarini R, Belli F, Parmiani G, Anichini A. Cytokine-mediated modulation of HLA-class II, ICAM-1, LFA-3, and tumor-associated antigen profile of melanoma cells. Comparison with anti-proliferative activity by rIL1-β, rTNF-α, rIFN-γ, rIL4 and their combinations. Int J Cancer 1990; 45:334-341.

94. Altomonte M, Gloghini A, Bertola G, Gasparollo A, Carbone A, Ferrone S, Maio M. Differential expression of cell adhesion molecules CD54/CD11a and CD58/CD2 by human melanoma cells and functional role in their interaction with cytotoxic cells. Cancer Res, In press.

95. Jonjic N, Alberti S, Bernasconi S, Peri G, Jilek P, Anichini A, Parmiani G, Mantovani A. Heterogeneous susceptibility of human melanoma clones to monocyte cytotoxicity: Role of ICAM-1 defined by antibody blocking and gene transfer. Eur J Immunol 1992; 22:2255-2260.

96. Becker JC, Dummer R, Hartmann AA, Burg G, Schmidt RE: Shedding of ICAM-1 from human melanoma cell lines induced by IFN-γ and tumor necrosis factor-α. J Immunol 1991; 147:4398-4401.

97. Lehmann JM, Holzmann B, Breitbart EW, Schmiegelow P, Riethmüller G, Johnson JP. Discrimination between benign and malignant cells of melanocytic lineage by two novel antigens, a glycoprotein with a molecular weight of 113,000 and a protein with a molecular weight of 76,000. Cancer Res 1987; 47:841-845.

98. Holzmann B, Bröcker EB, Lehmann JM, Ruiter DJ, Sorg C, Riethmüller G, Johnson JP. Tumor progression in human malignant melanoma: Five stages defined by either antigenic phenotypes. Int J Cancer 1987; 39:466-471.

99. Lehmann JM, Riethmüller G, Johnson JP. MUC18, a marker of tumor progression in human melanoma shows sequence similarity to the neural cell adhesion molecules of the immunoglobulin superfamily. Proc Natl Acad Sci USA 1989; 86:9891-9895.

100. Covault J. Molecular biology of cell adhesion in neural development. In: Glover DM and Hames BD, eds. Molecular Neurobiology. Oxford: IRL Press, 1989; pp 143-200.

101. Rutishauser U, Jessel TM. Cell adhesion molecules in vertebrate neural development. Physiol Rev 1988; 68:819-857.

102. Goridis C, Brunet J-F. NCAM: Structural diversity, function and regulation of expression. Cell Biol 1992; 3:189-197.

103. Pandolfi F, Trentin L, Boyle LA, Stamenkovic I, Byers R, Colvin RB, Kurnick JT. Expression of cell adhesion molecules in human melanoma cell lines and their role in cytotoxicity mediated by tumor-infiltrating lymphocytes. Cancer 1992; 69:1165-1173.

104. Denton KJ, Stretch JR, Gatter KC, Harris AL. A study of adhesion molecules as markers of progression in malignant melanoma. J Pathol 1992; 167:187-191.

105. Figarella-Branger DF, Durbec PL, Rougon GN. Differential spectrum of expression of neural cell adhesion molecule isoforms and L1 adhesion molecules on human neuroctodermal tumors. Cancer Res 1990; 50:6364-6370.

106. Wolff JM, Frank R, Mujoo K, Spiro RC, Reisfeld RA, Rathjen FG. A human brain glycoprotein related to the mouse cell adhesion molecule L1. J Biol Chem 1988; 263:11943-11947.

107. Harper JR, Prince JT, Healy PA, Stuark JK, Nauman SJ, Stallcup WB. Isolation and sequence of partial cDNA clones of human L1: Homology of human and rodent L1 in the cytoplasmic region. J Neurochem 1991; 56:797-804.

108. Jonjic N, Martin-Padura I, Pollicino T, Bernasconi S, Jilek P, Bigotti A, Mortarini R, Anichini A, Parmiani G, Colotta F, Dejana E, Mantovani A, Natali PG: Regulated expression of vascular cell adhesion molecule-1 in human malignant melanoma. Am J Pathol 1992; 141:1323-1330.

109. Williams AF, Barclay AN. The immunoglobulin superfamily-domains for cell surface recognition. Annu Rev Immunol 1988; 6:381-405.

110. Elices MJ, Osborn L, Takada Y, Crouse C, Luhowskyj S, Hemler ME, Lobb RR. VCAM-1 on activated endothelium interacts with the leukocyte integrin VLA-4 at a site distinct from the VLA-4/fibronectin binding site. Cell 1990; 60:577-584.

111. Benchimol S, Fuks A, Jothy S, Beauchemin N, Shirota K, Stanners CP. Carcinoembryonic antigen, a human tumor marker, functions as an intercellular adhesion molecule. Cell 1989; 57:327-334.

112. Oikawa S, Inuzuka C, Kuroki M, Matsuoka Y, Kosaki G, Nakazato H. Cell adhesion activity of non-specific cross-reacting antigen (NCA) and carcinoembryonic antigen (CEA) expressed on CHO cell surface: Homophilic and heterophilic adhesion. Biochem Biosphys Res Commun 1989; 164:39-45.

113. Wakabayashi S, Saito T, Shinohara N, Okamoto S, Tomioka H, Taniguchi M. Syn-

114. Dohi T, Nores G, Hakomori S. An IgG3 monoclonal antibody established after immunization with GM3 lactone: Immunochemical specificity and inhibition of melanoma cell growth in vitro and in vivo. Cancer Res 1988; 48:5680-5685.

geneic monoclonal antibodies against melanoma antigens with species specificity and interspecies crossreactivity. J Invest Dermatol 1984; 83:128-133.

115. Tai T, Ozawa H, Kawashima I. Generation of murine monoclonal antibodies specific for N-glycolylneuraminic acid-containing gangliosides. Arch Biochem Biophys 1992; 294:427-433.

116. Cahan LD, Irie RF, Singh R, Cassidenti A, Paulson JC. Identification of a human neuroectodermal tumor antigen (OFA-1-12) as ganglioside GD2. Proc Natl Acad Sci USA 1982; 79:7629-7633.

117. Cheresh DA, Pierschbacher MD, Herzig MA, Muggo K. Disialoganglioside GD2 and GD3 are involved in the attachment of human melanoma and neuroblastoma cells to extracellular matrix proteins. J Cell Biol 1986; 102:688-696.

118. Thurin J, Thurin M, Kimoto Y, Lubeck MD, Herlyn M, Elder DE, Smereczynska M, Karlsson KA, Clark WH Jr, Steplewski Z, Koprowski H: Monoclonal antibody-defined correlations in melanoma between levels of GD2 and GD3 antigens and antibody-mediated cytotoxicity. Cancer Res 1987; 47:1229-1233.

119. Cheung NK, Neely JE, Landmeier B, Nelson D, Miraldi F. Targeting of ganglioside GD2 monoclonal antibody to neuroblastoma. J Nucl Med 1987; 28:1577-1583.

120. Nudelman E, Hakomori S-I, Kannagi R, Levery S, Yeh M-Y, Hellström KE, Hellström I. Characterization of a human melanoma-associated ganglioside antigen defined by a monoclonal antibody, 4.2. J Biol Chem 1982; 257:12752-12756.

121. Dippold WG, Lloyd KO, Li LTC, Ideka H, Oettgen HF, Old LJ. Cell surface antigens of human malignant melanoma: Definition of six antigenic systems with mouse monoclonal antibodies. Proc Natl Acad Sci USA 1980; 77:6114-6118.

122. Pukel CS, Lloyd KO, Travassos LR, Dippold

WG, Oettgen HF, Old LJ. GD3—A prominent ganglioside of human melanoma: Detection and characterization by mouse monoclonal antibody. J Exp Med 1982; 155:1133-1147.

123. Hellström I, Brankovan V, Hellström KE. Strong antitumor activities with IgG3 antibodies to a human melanoma-associated ganglioside. Proc Natl Acad Sci USA 1985; 82:1499-1502.

124. Thurin J, Thurin M, Herlyn M, Elder DE, Steplewski Z, Clark WH Jr, Koprowski H. GD2 ganglioside biosynthesis is a distinct biochemical event in human melanoma tumor progression. FEBS Lett 1986; 208:17-22.

125. Natoli EJ Jr, Livingston PO, Pukel CS, Lloyd KO, Wiegandt H, Szalay J, Oettgen HF, Old LJ. A murine monoclonal antibody detecting N-acetyl-N-glycolyl-GM2: Characterization of cell surface activity. Cancer Res 1986; 46:4116-4120.

126. Cheresh DA, Reisfeld RA, Varki AP. O-acetylation of disialoganglioside GD3 by human melanoma cells creates a unique antigenic determinant. Science 1984; 225:844-846.

127. Cheresh DA, Varki AP, Varki NM, Stallup WB, Levine J, Reisfeld RA. A monoclonal antibody recognizes an O-acetylated sialic acid in a human melanoma-associated ganglioside. J Biol Chem 1984; 259:7453-7459.

128. Thurin J, Herlyn M, Hindsgaul O, Karlsson K-A, Stromberg N, Elder DE, Steplewski Z, Koprowski H. Proton NMR and fast atom bombardment mass spectrometry analysis of melanoma-associated ganglioside 9-O-acetyl-GD3. J Biol Chem 1985; 260:14556-14563.

129. Bernhard H, Roth S, Bauerschmitz J, Zum Büschenfeld K-HM, Dippold W. Immunorecognition of different ganglioside epitopes on human normal and melanoma tissues. Int J Cancer 1992; 51:568-572.

130. Lloyd KO, Gordon CM, Thampoe IJ, DiBenedetto C. Cell surface accessibility of individual gangliosides in malignant melanoma cells to antibodies is influenced by the total ganglioside composition of the cells. Cancer Res 1992; 52:4948-4953.

131. Tsuchida T, Saxton RE, Morton D, Irie RF. Gangliosides of human melanoma. Cancer 1989; 63:1166-1174.

132. Elder DE, Rodeck U, Thurin J, Cardillo F, Clark WH Jr, Stewart R, Herlyn M. Antigenic profile of tumor progression in human melanocytic nevi and melanomas. Cancer Res 1989; 49:5091-5096.

133. Iliopoulos D, Ernst C, Steplewski Z, Jambrosic JA, Rodeck U, Herlyn M, Clark WH Jr, Koprowski H, Herlyn D. Inhibition of metastases of a human melanoma xenograft by monoclonal antibody to the GD2/GD3 gangliosides. J Natl Cancer Inst 1989; 81:440-444.

134. Hersey P, Schibeci SD, Townsend P, Burns C, Cheresh D. Potentiation of lymphocyte response by monoclonal antibodies to the ganglioside GD3. Cancer Res 1986; 46:6083-6090.

135. Welte K, Miller G, Chapman PB, Yuas H, Natoli E, Kunicka JE, Cordon-Cardo C, Buhrer C, Old LJ, Houghton AN. Stimulation of T-lymphocyte proliferation by monoclonal antibodies against GD3 ganglioside. J Immunol 1987; 139:1763-1771.

136. Katoh-Semba R, Facci L, Skaper SD, Varon S. Gangliosides stimulate astroglial cell proliferation in the absence of serum. J Cell Physiol 1986; 126:147-153.

137. Natali PG, Bigotti A, Cavaliere R, Nicotra MR, Ferrone S. Phenotyping of lesions of melanocytic origin with monoclonal antibodies to melanoma-associated antigens and to the HLA-antigens. J Natl Cancer Inst 1984; 73:13-24.

138. Natali PG, Cordiali-Fei R, Cavaliere R, Pifilippo F, Quaranta V, Pellegrino MA, Ferrone S. Ia-like antigens on freshly explanted human melanoma. Clin Immunol Immunopathol 1981; 19:250-259.

139. Ruiter DJ, Bergman W, Welvarrt K, Scheffer E, van Vloten WA, Russo C, Ferrone S. Immunohistochemical analysis of malignant melanomas and nevocellular nevi with monoclonal antibodies to distinct monomorphic determinants of HLA antigens. Cancer Res 1984; 44:3930-3935.

140. Ruiter DJ, Bhan AK, Harris TJ, Sober AJ, Mihm MC Jr. Major histocompatibility antigens and mononuclear inflammatory infiltrate in benign nevomelanocytic proliferations and malignant melanoma. J Immunol 1982; 129:2808-2815.

141. Holzmann B, Broecker EB, Lehmann JM, Ruiter DJ, Sorg C, Riethmüller G, Johnson JP. Tumor progression in human malignant melanoma: Five stages determined by their antigenic phenotypes. Int J Cancer 1987; 39:466-471.

142. Van Duinen SG, Ruiter DJ, Broecker EB, van der Velde EA, Sorg C, Welvaart K, Ferrone S. Level of HLA antigens in locoregional metastases and clinical course of the disease in patients with melanoma. Cancer Res 1988; 48:1019-1025.

143. van Vreeswijk H, Ruiter DJ, Broecker EB, Welvaart K, Ferrone S. Differential expression of HLA-DR, -DQ, -DP antigens in primary and metastatic melanoma. J Invest Dermatol 1988; 90:755-760.

144. Versteeg R, Kruse-Wolters KM, Plomp AC, van Leeuwen AAD, Stam NJ, Pleogh HL, Ruiter DJ, Schrier PI. Suppression of class I human histocompatibility leukocyte antigen by c-*myc* is locus specific. J Exp Med 1989; 170:621-635.

145. Albino AP, Houghton AN, Eisinger M, Lee JS, Kantor RRS, Oliff AI, Old LJ. Class II major histocompatibility antigen expression in human melanocytes transformed by Harvey murine sarcoma virus (Ha-MSV) and Kirsten MSV (Ki-MSV) retroviruses. J Exp Med 1986; 164:1710-1722.

146. Crowley NJ, Darrow TL, Quinn-Allen M, Seigel HF. MHC-restricted recognition of autologous melanoma by tumor-specific cytotoxic T cells. J Immunol 1991; 146:1692-1699.

147. Pandolfi F, Boyle IA, Trentin L, Kurnick J, Isselbacher KJ, Gattoni-Celli S. Expression of HLA-A2 antigen in human melanoma cell lines and its role in T-cell recognition. Cancer Res 1991; 51:3164-3170.

148. Maio M, Altomonte M, Tatake R, Zeff RA, Ferrone S. Reduction in susceptibility to natural killer cell-mediated lysis of human FO-1 melanoma cells after induction of HLA class I antigen expression by transfection with B$_2$m gene. J Clin Invest 1991; 88:282-289.

149. Guerry D IV, Alexander MA, Herlyn M, Zehngebot LM, Mitchell KF, Zmijewski CM, Lusk EJ. HLA-DR histocompatibility leukocyte antigens permit cultured human melanoma cells from early but not advanced disease to stimulate autologous lymphocytes. J Clin Invest 1984; 73:267-271.

150. Fossati G, Taramelli D, Dalsari A, Bogdanovich G, Andreola S, Parmiani G. Primary but not metastatic human melanoma expressing DR antigens stimulate autologous lymphocytes. Int J Cancer 1984; 33:591-597.

151. Guerry D IV, Alexander MA, Elder DE, Herlyn M. Interferon-gamma regulated T-cell response to precursor nevi and biologically early melanoma. J Immunol 1987; 139:302-312.

152. Alexander M, Bennicelli J, Guerry D IV. Defective antigen presentation by human melanoma cell lines cultured from advanced, but not biologically early, disease. J Immunol 1989; 142:4070-4078.

153. Aaronson SA. Growth factors and cancer. Science 1992; 254:1146-1153.

154. Rodeck U, Herlyn M. Growth factors in melanoma. Cancer Met Rev 1991; 10:89-101.

155. Herlyn M, Malkowicz SB. Regulatory pathways in tumor growth and invasion. Lab Invest 1991; 65:262-271.

156. Rodeck U, Becker D, Herlyn M. Basic fibroblast growth factor in human melanoma. Cancer Cells 1991; 3:308-311.

157. Rodeck U, Melber K, Kath R, Herlyn M. Constitutive expression of multiple growth factor genes by melanoma cells but not normal melanocytes. J Invest Dermatol 1991; 97:20-26.

158. Armstrong CA, Tara DC, Hart CE, Köck A, Luger TA, Ansel JC. Heterogeneity of cytokine production by human malignant melanoma cells. Exp Dermatol 1992; 1:37-45.

159. Albino AP, Davis BM, Nanus DM. Induction of growth factor RNA expression in human malignant melanoma: Markers of transformation. Cancer Res 1991; 51:4815-4820.

160. Zachariae COC, Thestrup-Pedersen K, Matsushima K. Expression and secretion of leukocyte chemotactic cytokines by normal human melanocytes and melanoma cells. J Invest Dermatol 1991; 97:593-599.

161. Mattei S, Colombo MP, Melani C, Silvani A, Parmiani G, Herlyn M. Multichoice cytokine/growth factor and receptor loops in melanoma. Submitted.

162. Becker D, Meier CB, Herlyn M. Proliferation of human malignant melanomas is inhibited by antisense oligodeoxynucleotides targeted against basic fibroblast growth factor. EMBO J 1989; 8:3685-3691.

163. Halaban R, Kwon BS, Ghosh S, Delli-Bovi P, Baird A. Fibroblast growth factor as an autocrine growth factor for melanomas. Oncogene Res 1988; 3:177-186.

164. Kato J, Wanebo H, Calabresi P, Clark JW. Basic fibroblast growth factor production and growth factor receptors as potential targets for melanoma therapy. Melanoma Res 1992; 2:13-23.

165. Jaye M, Howk R, Burgess W, Ricca GA, Chiu I-M, Ravera MW, O'Brien SJ, Modi WS, Maciag T, Drohan WN. Human endothelial cell growth factor: Cloning, nucleotide sequence, and chromosome localization. Science 1986; 233:541-545.

166 Dickson C, Peters G. Potential oncogene product related to growth factors. Science 1987; 326:833.

167. Delli-Bovi P, Curatola AM, Kern FG, Greco A, Ittmann M, Basilico C. An oncogene isolated by transfection of Kaposi's sarcoma DNA encodes a growth factor that is a member of FGF family. Cell 1987; 50:729-737.

168. Zhan X, Bates B, Hu X, Goldfarb M. The human FGF-5 oncogene encodes a novel protein related to fibroblast growth factors. Mol Cell Biol 1988; 8:3487-3495.

169. Marics I, Adelaide J, Raybaud F, Mattei M-G, Coulier F, Planche J, de Lapeyriere O, Birnbaum D. Characterization of the *HST*-related *FGF6* gene, a new member of the fibroblast growth factor family. Oncogene 1989; 4:335-340.

170. Finch PW, Rubin JS, Miki T, Ron D, Aaronson SA. Human KGF is FGF-related with properties of a paracrine effector of epithelial cell growth. Science 1989; 245:752-755.

171. Abraham JA, Whang JL, Tumolo A, Mergia A, Friedman J, Gospodarowicz D, Fiddes JC. Human basic fibroblast growth factor: Nucleotide sequence and genomic organization. EMBO J 1986; 5:2523-2528.

172. Shing Y, Folkman J, Sullivan R, Butterfield C, Murray J, Klagsbrun M. Heparin-affinity: Purification of a tumor-derived capillary endothelial cell growth factor. Science 1984; 223:1296-1299.

173. Zhu X, Komiya H, Chirino A, Faham S, Fox GM, Arakawa T, Hsu BT, Rees DC. Three-dimensional structures of acidic and basic fibroblast growth factors. Science 1991; 251:90-93.

174. Cordon-Cardo C, Vlodavsky I, Haimovitz-Friedman A, Hicklin D, Fuks Z. Expression of basic fibroblast growth factor in normal human tissues. Lab Invest 1990; 63:832-840.

175. Schulze-Osthoff K, Risau W, Vollmer E, Sorg C. In situ detection of basic fibroblast growth factors by highly specific antibodies. Am J Pathol 1990; 137:85-92.

176. Zagzag D, Miller DC, Sato Y, Rifkin DB, Burnstein DE. Immunohistochemical localization of basic fibroblast growth factor in astrocytomas. Cancer Res 1990; 50:7393-7398.

177. Takahashi JA, Mori H, Fukumoto M, Igarashi K, Jaye M, Oda Y, Kikuchi H, Hatanaka M. Gene expression of fibroblast growth factors in human gliomas and meningiomas: Demonstration of cellular source of basic fibroblast growth factor mRNA and peptide in human tissues. Proc Natl Acad Sci USA 1990; 87:5710-5714.

178. Scott G, Stoler M, Sarkar S, Halaban R. Localization of basic fibroblast growth factor mRNA in melanocytic lesions by in situ hybridization. J Invest Dermatol 1991; 96:318-322.

179. Mancianti ML, Györfi T, Shih I-M, Levengood G, Valyi-Nagy I, Menssen H-D, Halpern AC, Elder DE, Herlyn M. Growth regulation of cultured human nevus cells. J Invest Dermatol 1993; In press.

180. Morrison RS. Suppression of basic fibroblast growth factor expression by antisense oligodeoxynucleotides inhibits growth of transformed human astrocytes. J Biol Chem 1991; 266:728-734.

181. Corin SJ, Chen LC, Hamburger AW. Enhancement of anchorage-independent growth of a human adrenal carcinoma cell line by endogenously produced basic fibroblast growth factor. Int J Cancer 1990; 46:516-521.

182. Montesano R, Vassalli J-D, Baird A, Guillemin R, Orci L. bFGF induces angiogenesis in vitro. Proc Natl Acad Sci USA 1986; 83:7297-7301.

183. Tsuboi R, Sato Y, Rifkin DB. Correlation of cell migration, cell invasion, receptor number, proteinase production, and basic fibroblast growth factor levels in endothelial cells. J Cell Biol 1990; 110:511-517.

184. Goldfarb M. The fibroblast growth factor family. Cell Growth Diff 1990; 1:439-445.

185. Vlodavsky I, Folkman R, Sullivan R, Friedman R, Ishai-Michaeli R, Sasse J, Klagsbrun M. Endothelial cell-derived basic fibroblast growth factor synthesis and deposition into subendothelial extracellular matrix. Proc Natl Acad Sci USA 1987; 84:2292-2296.

186. Saksela O, Rifkin DB. Release of bFGF-heparan sulfate complexes from endothelial cells by PA-mediated proteolytic activity. J Cell Biol 1990; 110:767-775.

187. Kandel J, Bossy-Wetzel E, Radvanyl F, Klagsbrun M, Folkman J, Hanahan D. Neovascularization is associated with a switch to the export of bFGF in the multistep development of fibrosarcoma. Cell 1991; 66:1095-1104.

188. Presta M, Maier JAM, Rusnati M, Ragnotti G. bFGF is released from endothelial ECM in a biologically active form. J Cell Physiol 1989; 140:68-74.

189. Buckley-Sturrock A, Woodward SC, Senior RM, Griffin GL, Klagsbrun M, Davidson JM. Differential stimulation of collagenase and chemotactic activity in fibroblasts derived from rat wound repair tissue and human skin by growth factors. J Cell Physiol 1989; 138:70-78.

190. Klagsbrun M, Baird A. A dual receptor system is required for basic fibroblast growth factor activity. Cell 1991; 67:229-231.

191. Becker D, Lee PL, Rodeck U, Herlyn M. Inhibition of the fibroblast growth factor receptor 1 (FGFR-1) gene in human melanocytes and malignant melanomas leads to inhibition of proliferation and signs indicative of differentiation. Oncogene 1992; 7:2303-2313.

192. Adelaide J, Mattei M-G, Marics I, Raybaud F, Planche J, de Lapeyriere O, Birnbaum D. Chromosomal localization of the *hst* oncogene and its co-amplification with the *int.2* oncogene in a human melanoma. Oncogene 1988; 2:413-416.

193. Theillet C, Le Roy X, de Lapeyriere O, Grosgeorges J, Adnane J, Raynaud SD, Simony-Lafontaine J, Goldfarb M, Escot C, Birnbaum D, Gaudray P. Amplification of *FGF*-related genes in human tumors: Possible involvement of *HST* in breast carcinomas. Oncogene 1989; 4:915-922.

194. Derynck R. Transforming growth factor alpha. Cell 1988; 54:593-595.

195. Derynck R, Roberts AB, Winkler ME, Chen EY, Goeddel DV. Human transforming growth factor-α: Precursor structure and expression in *E. coli*. Cell 1984; 38:287-297.

196. Todaro GJ, Fryling C, DeLarco JE. Transforming growth factors produced by certain human tumor cells: Polypeptides that interact with epidermal growth factor receptors. Proc Natl Acad Sci USA 1980; 77:5258-5262.

197. Marquardt H, Todaro G. Human transforming growth factor production by a melanoma cell line, purification, and initial characterization. J Biol Chem 1982; 257:5220-5225.

198. DeLarco JE, Pigott DA, Lazarus JA. Ectopic peptides released by a human melanoma cell line that modulate the transformed phenotype. Proc Natl Acad Sci USA 1985; 82:5015-5019.

199. Imanishi K, Yamaguchi K, Suzuki M, Honda S, Yanaihara N, Abe K. Production of transforming growth factor-α in human tumor cell lines. Br J Cancer 1989; 59:761-765.

200. Inagaki H, Katoh M, Kurosawa-Ohsawa K, Tanaka S. A new sandwich enzyme-linked immunosorbent assay (ELISA) for transforming growth factor alpha (TGF-α) based upon conformational modification by antibody binding. J Immunol Meth 1990; 128:27-37.

201. Kim MK, Warren TC, Kimball ES. Purification and characterization of a low molecular weight transforming growth factor from the urine of melanoma patients. J Biol Chem 1985; 260:9237-9243.

202. Ellis DL, Chow JC, King LE. Detection of urinary TGF-α by HPLC and Western blot in patients with melanoma. J Invest Dermatol 1990; 95:27-30.

203. Hudgins WR, Orth DN, Stromberg K. Variant forms of rat epidermal growth factor present in the urine of nude rats bearing human tumors. Cancer Res 1988; 48:1428-1434.

204. Derynck R, Goeddel DV, Ullrich A, Gutterman JU, Williams RD, Bringman TS, Berger WH. Synthesis of messenger RNAs for transforming growth factors alpha and

beta and the epidermal growth factor receptor by human tumors. Cancer Res 1987; 47:702-712.

205. Lizonova A, Bizik J, Grofova M, Vaheri A. Coexpression of tumor-associated α2-macroglobulin and growth factors in human melanoma cells. J Cell Biochem 1990; 43:315-323.

206. Ellem KA, Cullinan M, Baumann KC, Dunstan A. UVR induction of TGF-α: A possible autocrine mechanism for the melanocytic response and for promotion of epidermal carcinogenesis. Carcinogenesis 1988; 9:797-801.

207. Chenevix-Trench G, Cullinan M, Ellem KAO, Hayward NK. UV induction of transforming growth factor α in melanoma cell lines is a posttranslational event. J Cell Physiol 1992; 152:328-336.

208. Koprowski H, Herlyn M, Balaban G, Parmiter A, Ross A, Nowell P. Expression of the receptor for epidermal growth factor correlates with increased dosage of chromosome 7 in malignant melanomas. Somat Cell Mol Genet 1985; 11:297-302.

209. Real FX, Rettig WJ, Chesa PG, Melamed MR, Old LJ, Mendelsohn J. Expression of epidermal growth factor receptor in human cultured cells and tissues: Relationship to cell lineage and stage of differentiation. Cancer Res 1986; 46:4726-4731.

210. Elder DE, Rodeck U, Thurin J, Cardillo F, Clark WH Jr, Stewart R, Herlyn M. Antigenic profile of tumor progression in human melanocytic nevi and melanomas. Cancer Res 1989; 49:5091-5096.

211. de Wit PEJ, Moretti S, Koenders PG, Weterman MAJ, van Muijen GNP, Gianotti B, Ruiter DJ. Increasing epidermal growth factor receptor expression in human melanocytic tumor progression. J Invest Dermatol 1992; 99:168-173.

212. Rodeck U, Herlyn M, Menssen HD, Furlanetto RW, Koprowski H. Metastatic but not primary melanoma cells grow in vitro independently of exogenous growth factors. Int J Cancer 1987; 40:687-690.

213. Sauvagio S, Fretts RE, Riopelle RJ, Lagarde AE. Autonomous proliferation of MeWo human melanoma cell lines in serum-free medium: Secretion of growth-stimulating activities. Int J Cancer 1986; 37:123-132.

214. Singletary SE, Baker FL, Spitzer G, Tucker SL, Tomasovic B, Brock WA, Ajani JA, Kelly AM. Biologic effect of epidermal growth factor on the in vitro growth of human tumors. Cancer Res 1987; 47:403-406.

215. Herlyn M, Mancianti M-L, Jambrosic J, Bolen JB, Koprowski H. Regulatory factors that determine growth and phenotype of normal human melanocytes. Exp Cell Res 1988; 179:322-331.

216. Rodeck U, Williams N, Murthy U, Herlyn M. Monoclonal antibody 425 inhibits growth stimulation of carcinoma cells by exogenous EGF and tumor-derived TGF-α. J Cell Biochem 1990; 10:69-80.

217. Kudlow JE, Khosravi MJ, Kobrin MS, Mak WW. Inability of an anti-epidermal growth factor receptor monoclonal antibody to block 'autocrine' growth stimulation in transforming growth factor-secreting melanoma cells. J Biol Chem 1984; 259:11895-11900.

218. Massagué J. The transforming growth factor-beta family. Ann Rev Cell Biol 1990; 6:597-641.

219. Valverius EM, Walker-Jones D, Bates SE, Stampfer MR, Clark R, McCormick F, Dickson RB, Lippmann ME. Production of and responsiveness to transforming growth factor-β in normal and oncogene-transformed human mammary epithelial cells. Cancer Res 1989; 49:6269-6274.

220. Arteaga CL, Coffey RJ, Dugger TC, McCutchen CM, Moses HL, Lyons RM. Growth stimulation of human breast cancer cells with anti-transforming growth factor β antibodies: Evidence for negative autocrine regulation by transforming growth factor β. Cell Growth Diff 1990; 1:367-374.

221 Pittelkow MR, Shipley GD. Serum-free culture of normal human melanocytes: Growth kinetics, and growth factor requirements. J Cell Physiol 1989; 140:565-576.

222. Rodeck U, Melber K, Kath R, Menssen H-D, Varello M, Atkinson B, Herlyn M. Constitutive expression of multiple growth factor genes by melanoma cells but not normal melanocytes. J Invest Dermatol 1991; 97:20-26.

223. Lizonova A, Bizik J, Grofova M, Vaheri A. Coexpression of tumor-associated α2-macroglobulin and growth factors in human melanoma cells. J Cell Biochem 1990; 43:315-323.

224. Bodmer S, Strommer K, Frei K, Siepl C, deTribolet N, Heid I, Fontana A. Immunosuppression and transforming growth factor-β in glioblastoma: Preferential production of transforming growth factor-β_2. J Immunol 1989; 143:3222-3229.

225. DeLarco JE, Pigott DA, Lazarus JA. Ectopic peptides released by a human melanoma cell line that modulate the transformed phenotype. Proc Natl Acad Sci USA 1985; 82:5015-5019.

226. Albino AP, Davis BM, Nanus DM. Induction of growth factor RNA expression in human malignant melanoma: Markers of transformation. Cancer Res 1991; 51:4815-4820.

227. Herlyn M, Malkowicz SB. Regulatory pathways in tumor growth and invasion. Lab Invest 1991; 65:262-271.

228. Massagué J. Receptors of the TGF-β family. Cell 1992; 69:1067-1070.

229. Heldin C-H, Westermark B. Platelet-derived growth factor: Mechanism of action and possible in vivo function. Cell Regulation 1990; 1:555-566.

230. Johnsson A, Heldin C-H, Wasteson A, Westermark B, Deuel TF, Huang JS, Seeburg PH, Gray A, Ullrich A, Scrace G, Stroobant P, Waterfield MD. The c-sis gene encodes a precursor of the B chain of platelet-derived growth factor. EMBO J 1984; 3:921-928.

231. Waterfield MD, Scarce GT, Whittle N, Stroobant P, Phonsson A, Wasteson A, Westermark B, Heldin C-H, Huang JS, Deuel TF. Platelet-derived growth factor is structurally related to the putative transforming protein p28 sis of simian sarcoma virus. Nature 1983; 304:35-39.

232. Leal F, Williams LT, Robbins KC, Aaronsson SA. Evidence that the v-sis gene product transforms by interaction with the receptor for platelet-derived growth factor. Science 1985; 230:327-330.

233. Johnsson A, Betsholtz C, Heldin C-H, Westermark B. Antibodies against platelet-derived growth factor inhibit acute transformation by simian sarcoma virus. Nature 1985; 317:438-440.

234. Westermark B, Johnsson A, Paulsson Y, Betsholtz C, Heldin C-H, Herlyn M, Rodeck U, Koprowski H. Human melanoma cell lines of primary and metastatic origin express the genes encoding the chains of platelet-derived growth factor. Proc Natl Acad Sci USA 1987; 83:7197-7200.

235. Lizonova A, Bizik J, Grofova M, Vaheri A. Coexpression of tumor-associated α_2-macroglobulin and growth factors in human melanoma cells. J Cell Biochem 1990; 43:315-323.

236. Chenevix-Trent G, Martin NG, Ellem KA. Gene expression in melanoma cell lines and cultured melanocytes: correlation between levels of c-src-1, c-myc, and p53. Cancer Res 1990; 50:1190-1193.

237. Rakowicz-Szulczynska EM, Rodeck U, Herlyn M, Koprowski H. Chromatin binding of EGF, NGF, and PDGF in cells bearing the appropriate surface receptors. Proc Natl Acad Sci USA 1987; 83:3728-3732.

238. Rakowicz-Szulczynska EM, Koprowski H. Antagonistic effect of PDGF and NGF on transcription of ribosomal DNA and tumor cell proliferation. Biochem Biophys Res Commun 1989; 163:649-656.

239. Harsh GR, Keating MT, Escobedo JA, Williams LT. Platelet derived growth factor (PDGF) autocrine components in human tumor cell lines. J Neurooncol 1990; 8:1-12.

240. Keating MT, Williams LT. Autocrine stimulation of intracellular PDGF receptors in v-sis-transformed cells. Science 1988; 239:914-916.

241. Forsberg K, Valyi-Nagy I, Heldin C-H, Herlyn M, Westermark B. Platelet-derived growth factor (PDGF) in oncogenesis: development of a vascular connective tissue stroma in xenotransplanted human melanoma producing PDGF-BB. Proc Natl Acad Sci USA 1992; 90:393-397.

242. Hartmann N, Fang W, Herlyn M, Rodeck U, Wellstein A. Pentosanpolysulfate inhibits heparin-binding growth factor activity from melanoma in vitro and reduces melanoma growth and metastases in nude mice. Submitted.

243. Li Y-S, Milner PG, Chauhan AK, Watson MA, Hoffman RM, Kodner CM, Milbrandt J, Deuel TF. Cloning and expression of a developmentally regulated protein that induces mitogenic and neurite outgrowth activity. Science 1990; 250:1690-1694.

244. Böhlen P, Müller T, Gautschi-Sova P, Albrecht U, Rasool CG, Decker M, Seddon A, Fafeur V, Kovesdi I, Kretschmer P. Isolation from bovine

brain and structural characterization of HBN, a heparin-binding neurotrophic factor. Growth Factors 1991; 4:97-107.

245. Lai S, Czubayko F, Riegel AT, Wellstein A. Structure of the human heparin-binding growth factor gene pleiotrophin. Biochem Biophys Res Commun 1992; 187:1113-1122.

246. Merenmies J, Rauvala H. Molecular cloning of the 18-kDa growth-associated protein of developing brain. J Biol Chem 1990; 265:16721-16724.

247. Wellstein A, Fang W, Khatri A, Lu Y, Swain SS, Dickson RB, Sasse J, Tate Riegel A, Lippman ME. A heparin-binding growth factor secreted from breast cancer cells homologous to a developmentally regulated cytokine. J Biol Chem 1992; 267:2582-2587.

248. Richmond A, Balentien E, Thomas HG, Flaggs G, Barton DE, Spiess J, Bordoni R, Franke U, Derynck R. Molecular characterization and chromosomal mapping of melanoma growth stimulatory activity, a growth factor structurally related to beta-thromboglobulin. EMBO J 1988; 7:2025-2033.

249. Wolpe SD, Cerami A. Macrophage inflammatory proteins 1 and 2: members of a novel superfamily of cytokines. FASEB J 1989; 3:2565-2573.

250. Richmond A, Thomas HG. Purification of melanoma growth stimulatory activity. J Cell Physiol 1986; 129:375-384.

251. Schröder JM, Persoon NL, Christophers E. Lipopolysaccharide-stimulated monocytes secrete, apart from neutrophil-activating peptide 1/interleukin 8, a second neutrophil-activating protein. NH2-terminal amino acid sequence identity with melanoma growth stimulatory activity. J Exp Med 1990; 171:1091-1100.

252. Moser B, Clark-Lewis I, Zwahlen R, Baggilioni M. Neutrophil-activating properties of the melanoma growth-stimulatory activity. J Exp Med 1990; 171:1797-1802.

253. Richmond A, Lawson DH, Nixon DW, Stedman NJ, Stevens S, Chawla RK. Extraction of a melanoma-growth stimulatory activity from culture medium conditioned by the Hs0294T human melanoma cell line. Cancer Res 1983; 43:2106-2112.

254. Richmond A, Lawson DH, Nixon DW, Chawla RK. Characterization of auto-

stimulatory and transforming growth factors from human melanoma cells. Cancer Res 1985; 45:6390-6394.

255. Lawson DH, Thomas HG, Roy RGB, Gordon DS, Chawla RK, Nixon DW, Richmond A. Preparation of a monoclonal antibody to melanoma growth-stimulatory activity released into serum-free culture medium by Hs0294T malignant melanoma cells. J Cell Biochem 1987; 34:169-185.

256. Bordoni R, Thomas G, Richmond A. Growth factor modulation of melanoma-growth stimulatory activity mRNA expression in human malignant melanoma cells correlates well with cell growth. J Cell Biochem 1989; 39:421-428.

257. Rodeck U, Melber K, Kath R, Herlyn M. Constitutive expression of multiple growth factor genes by melanoma cells but not normal melanocytes. J Invest Dermatol 1991; 97:20-26.

258. Chenevix-Trent G, Martin NG, Ellem KA. Gene expression in melanona cell lines and cultured melanocytes: correlation between levels of c-*src*-1, c-*myc*, and p53. Cancer Res 1990; 50:1190-1193.

259. Moser B, Schumacher C, von-Tscharner V, Clark-Lewis I, Baggiolini M. Neutrophil-activating peptide 2 and gro/melanoma growth-stimulatory activity interact with neutrophil-activating peptide 1/interleukin 8 receptors on human neutrophils. J Biol Chem 1991; 266:10666-10671.

260. Cheng QC, Han JH, Thomas HG, Balentien E, Richmond A. The melanoma growth stimulatory activity receptor consists of two proteins. Ligand binding results in enhanced tyrosine phosphorylation. J Immunol 1992; 148:451-456.

261. Horuk R, Yansura DG, Reilly D, Spencer S, Bourell J, Henzel W, Rice G, Unemori E. Purification, receptor binding analysis, and biological characterization of human melanoma growth stimulating activity (MGSA). Evidence for a novel MGSA receptor. J Biol Chem 1993; 268:541-546.

262. Strieter RM, Kasahara K, Allen RM, Standiford TJ, Rolfe MW, Becker FS, Chensue SW, Kunkel SL. Cytokine-induced neutrophil-derived interleukin-8. Am J Pathol 1992; 141:397-407.

263. Wang JM, Taraboletti G, Matsushima K, Van Damme J, Mantovani A. Induction of haptotactic migration of melanoma cells by neutrophil activating protein/interleukin-8. Biochem Biophys Res Commun 1990; 169:165-170.

264. Van Meir E, Ceska M, Effenberger F, Walz A, Grouzmann E, Desbaillets I, Frei K, Fontana A, de Tribolet N. Interleukin-8 is produced in neoplastic and infectious diseases of the human central nervous system. Cancer Res 1992; 52:4297-4305.

265. Tuschil A, Lam C, Haslberger A, Lindley I. Interleukin-8 stimulates calcium transiently and promotes epidermal cell proliferation. J Invest Dermatol 1992; 99:294-298.

266. Smoller BR, Krueger J. Detection of cytokine-induced protein γ-immune protein-10 (γ-IP10) in atypical melanocytic proliferations. J Am Acad Dermatol 1991; 25:627-631.

267. Unemori EN, Amento EP, Bauer EA, Horuk R. Melanoma growth-stimulatory activity/GRO decreases collagen expression by human fibroblasts. Regulation by C-X-C but not C-C cytokines. J Biol Chem 1993; 268:1338-1342.

268. Gery I, Waksman BH. Potentiation of the T-lymphocytic response to mitogens. II. The cellular source of potentiating mediator(s). J Exp Med 1972; 136:143-155.

269. di Giovine FS, Duff GW. Interleukin 1: the first interleukin. Immunol Today 1990; 11:13-20.

270. Onozaki K, Matsushima K, Aggarwal BB, Oppenheim JJ. Human interleukin 1 is a cytocidal factor for several tumor cell lines. J Immunol 1985; 135:3962-3968.

271. Nakai S, Mizuno K, Kaneta M, Hirai Y. A simple, sensitive bioassay for the detection of interleukin-1 using the human melanoma A375 cell line. Biochem Biophys Res Commun 1988; 154:1189-1196.

272. Mortarini R, Belli F, Parmiani G, Anichini A. Cytokine-mediated modulation of HLA-class II, INCAM, LFA-3 and tumor-associated antigen profile of melanoma cells. Int J Cancer 1990; 45:334-341.

273. Giavazzi R, Garofalo A, Banie MR, Abbate M, Ghezzi P, Boraschi D, Mantovani A, Dejana E. Interleukin 1 induced augmentation of experimental metastases from a human melanoma in nude mice. Cancer Res 1990; 50:4771-4775.

274. Köck A, Schwarz T, Urbanski A, Peng Z, Vetterlein M, Miksche M, Ansel JC, Kung HF, Luger TA. Expression and release of interleukin-1 by different human melanoma cell lines. J Natl Cancer Inst 1988; 81:36-42.

275. Bennicelli JL, Elias J, Kern J, Guerry D IV. Production of interleukin 1 activity by cultured human melanoma cells. Cancer Res 1989; 49:930-935.

276. Colombo MP, Maccalli C, Mattei S, Melani C, Radrizzani M, Parmiani G. Expression of cytokine genes, including IL-6, in human malignant melanoma cell lines. Melanoma Res 1992; 2:181-189.

277. Rice EG, Bevilacqua M. An inducible endothelial cell surface glycoprotein mediates melanoma adhesion. Science 1989; 246:1303-1306.

278. Shabon U, Bennicelli JL, Guerry D IV, Koprowski H, Ricciardi RP. Human melanoma cells transcribe interleukin 1 genes identical to those of monocytes. Cancer Res 1991; 51:3334-3335.

279. Burrow FJ, Haskard DO, Hart IR, Marshall JF, Selkirk S, Poole S, Thorpe PE. Influence of tumor-derived interleukin 1 on melanoma-endothelial cell interactions in vitro. Cancer Res 1991; 51:4768-4775.

280. Cornil I, Theodorescu D, Mau S, Herlyn M, Jambrosic J, Kerbel RS. Fibroblast cell interactions with human melanoma cells affect tumor cell growth as a function of tumor progression. Proc Natl Acad Sci USA 1991; 88:6028-6032.

281. Lu C, Vickers MF, Kerbel RS. Interleukin 6: A fibroblast-derived growth inhibitor of human melanoma cells from early but not advanced stages of tumor progression. Proc Natl Acad Sci USA 1992; 89:9215-9219.

282. Lu C, Kerbel RS. Interleukin 6: transition from paracrine growth inhibitor to intracellular autocrine stimulator during human melanoma progression. J Cell Biol 1992; 120:1281-1288.

283. Swope VB, Abdel-Malek Z, Kassem LM, Nordlund JJ. Interleukins 1α and 6 and tumor necrosis factor-α are paracrine inhibitors of human melanocyte proliferation and melanogenesis. J Invest Dermatol 1991; 96:180-185.

284. Armstrong CA, Tara DC, Hart CE, Köck A, Luger TA, Ansel JC. Heterogeneity of cytokine production by human malignant melanoma cells. Exp Dermatol 1992; 1:37-45.

285. Kishimoto T, Akira S, Taga T. Interleukin-6 and its receptor: A paradigm for cytokines. Science 1992; 258:593-597.

286. Ip NY, Nye SH, Boulton TG, Davis S, Taga T, Li Y, Birren SJ, Yasukawa K, Kishimoto T, Anderson DJ, Stahl N, Yancopoulos GD. CNTF and LIF act on neuronal cells via shared signaling pathways that involve the IL-6 signal transducing receptor component gp130. Cell 1992; 69:1121-1132.

287. Gearing DP, Comeau MR, Friend DJ, Gimpel SD, Thut CJ, McGourty J, Brasher KK, King JA, Gillis S, Mosley B, Ziegler SF, Cosman D: The IL-6 signal transducer, gp130: An oncostatin M receptor and affinity converter for the LIF receptor. Science 1992; 255:1434-1437.

288. Mattei S, Colombo MP, Melani C, Silvani A, Parmiani G, Herlyn M. Multichoice cytokine-growth factor and receptor loops in melanoma. Submitted.

289. Mori M, Yamaguchi K, Honda S, Nagasaki K, Ueda M, Abe O, Abe K. Cancer cachexia syndrome developed in nude mice bearing melanoma cells producing leukemia-inhibitory factor. Cancer Res 1991; 51:6656-6659.

290. Rodeck U, Herlyn M, Menssen HD, Furlanetto RW, Koprowski H. Metastatic but not primary melanoma cells grow in vitro independently of exogenous growth factors. Int J Cancer 1987; 40:687-690.

291. Rodeck U, Melber K, Kath R, Herlyn M. Constitutive expression of multiple growth factor genes by melanoma cells but not normal melanocytes. J Invest Dermatol 1991; 97:20-26.

292. Stracke ML, Engel JD, Wilson LW, Rechler MM, Liotta LA, Schiffman E. The type I insulin-like growth factor receptor is a motility receptor in human melanoma cells. J Biol Chem 1989; 264:21544-21549.

293. Stracke ML, Kohn EC, Aznavoorian SA, Wilson LL, Salomon D, Krutzch HC, Liotta LA, Schiffman E. Insulin-like growth factors stimulate chemotaxis in human melanoma cells. Biochem Biophys Res Commun 1988; 153:1076-1083.

294. Furlong RA. The biology of hepatocyte growth factor/scatter factor. BioEssays 1992; 14:613-617.

295. Prat M, Narsimhan RP, Crepaldi T, Nicotra MR, Natali PG, Comoglio PM. The receptor encoded by the human c-*met* oncogene is expressed in hepatocytes, epithelial cells and solid tumors. Int J Cancer 1991; 49:323-328.

296. Halaban R, Rubin JS, Funasaka Y, Cobb M, Boulton T, Faletto D, Rosen E, Chan A, Yoko K, White W, Cook C, Moellmann G. *Met* and hepatocyte growth factor/scatter factor signal transduction in normal melanocytes and melanoma cells. Oncogene 1992; 7:2195-2206.

297. Walker MJ. Role of hormones and growth factors in melanomas. Sem Oncol 1988; 15:512-523.

298. Ghanem GE, Comunale G, Libert A, Vercammen-Grandjean A, Lejeune FJ. Evidence for α-melanocyte-stimulating hormone (α-MSH) receptors on human melanoma cells. Int J Cancer 1988; 41:248-255.

299. Siegrist W, Solca F, Stutz S, Giuffre S, Carrel J, Girard J, Eberle AN. Characterization of receptors for α-melanocyte-stimulating hormone on human melanoma cells. Cancer Res 1989; 49:6352-6358.

300. Tatro JB, Atkins M, Mier JW, Hardarson S, Wolfe H, Smith T, Entwistle ML, Reichlin S. Melanotropin receptors demonstrated in situ in human melanoma. J Clin Invest 1990; 85:1825-1832.

301. Ghanem G, Verstegen J, Liberat A, Arnould R, Lejeune F. α-melanocyte-stimulating hormone immunoreactivity in human melanoma metastases extracts. Pigment Cell Res 1989; 2:519-523.

302. Ellem KA, Kay GF. The nature of conditioning nutrients for malignant melanoma cultures. J Cell Sci 1983; 62:249-266.

303. Lerner AB, McGuire JS. Melanocyte stimulating hormone and adrenocorticotropic hormone: their relationship to pigmentation. N Engl J Med 1964; 270:539-546.

304. Fuller BB, Meyskens FL. Endocrine responsiveness in human melanocytes and melanoma cells in culture. J Natl Cancer Inst 1981; 66:799-802.

305. Mountjoy KG, Robbins LS, Mortrud MT, Cone RD. The cloning of a family of genes that encode the melanocortin receptors. Science 1992; 257:1248-1251.

306. Chhajlani V, Wikberg JES. Molecular cloning and expression of the human melanocyte stimulating hormone receptor cDNA. FEBS Lett 1992; 309:417-420.

307. Heldin C-H, Usuki K, Miyazono K. Platelet-derived endothelial cell growth factor. J Cell Biochem 1991; 47:208-210.

308. Ferrara N, Houck KA, Jakeman LB, Winer J, Leung DW. The vascular endothelial growth factor family of polypeptides. J Cell Biochem 1991; 47:211-218.

309. Gitay-Goren H, Halaban R, Neufeld G. Human melanoma cells but not normal melanocytes express vascular endothelial growth factor receptors. Biochem Biophys Res Commun 1993; 190:702-709.

310. Bogdahn U, Apfel R, Hahn M, Gerlach M, Behl C, Hoppe J, Martin R. Autocrine tumor cell growth-inhibiting activities from human malignant melanoma. Cancer Res 1989; 49:5358-5363.

311. Weilbach FX, Bogdahn U, Poot M, Apfel R, Behl C, Drenkard D, Martin R, Hoehn H. Melanoma-inhibiting activity inhibits cell proliferation by prolongation of the S-phase and arrest of cells in the G2 compartment. Cancer Res 1990; 50:6981-6986.

312. Apfel R, Lottspeich F, Hoppe J, Behl C, Dürr G, Bogdahn U. Purification and analysis of growth regulating proteins secreted by a human melanoma cell line. Melanoma Res 1992; 2:327-336.

313. Lu C, Vickers MF, Kerbel RS. Interleukin 6: a fibroblast-derived growth inhibitor of human melanoma cells from early but not advanced stages of tumor progression. Proc Natl Acad Sci USA 1992; 89:9215-9219.

314. Johns TG, Mackay IR, Callister KA, Hertzog PJ, Devenish RJ, Linnane AW. Antiproliferative potencies of interferons on melanoma cell lines and xenografts: Higher efficacy of interferon β. J Natl Cancer Inst 1992; 84:1185-1190.

315 Parry RL, Chin T, Epstein J, Hudson PL, Powell DM, Donahoe PK. Recombinant human Mullerian inhibiting substance inhibits human ocular melanoma cell lines in vitro and in vivo. Cancer Res 1992; 52:1182-1186.

316. Yarden Y, Ullrich A. Growth factor receptor tyrosine kinases. Ann Rev Biochem 1988; 57:443-478.

317. Schlessinger J, Ullrich A. Growth factor signaling by receptor tyrosine kinases. Neuron 1992; 9:383-391.

318. Easty DJ, Ganz SE, Farr CJ, Lai C, Herlyn M, Bennett DC. Novel and known protein tyrosine kinases and their abnormal expression in human melanoma. Submitted.

319. Becker D, Beebe SJ, Herlyn M. Differential expression of protein kinase C and cAMP-dependent protein kinase in normal human melanocytes and malignant melanomas. Oncogene 1990; 5:1133-1139.

320. Yamanishi DT, Graham M, Buckmeier JA, Meyskens FL Jr. The differential expression of protein kinase C genes in normal human neonatal melanocytes and metastatic melanomas. Carcinogenesis 1991; 12:105-109.

321. Arita Y, O'Driscoll KR, Weinstein IB. Growth of human melanocyte cultures supported by 12-O-tetradecanoylphorbol-13-acetate is mediated through protein kinase C activation. Cancer Res 1992; 52:4514-4521.

322. Coppock DL, Tansey JB, Nathanson L. 12-O-tetradecanoylphorbol-13-acetate induces transient cell cycle arresting G1 and G2 in metastatic melanoma cells: inhibition of phosphorylation of p34cdc^2. Cell Growth Diff 1992; 3:485-494.

323. Gruber JR, Ohno S, Niles RM. Increased expression of protein kinase Ca plays a key role in retinoic acid-induced melanoma differentiation. J Biol Chem 1992; 267:13356-13360.

324. Moore BW. A soluble protein characteristic of the nervous system. Biochem Biophys Res Commun 1965; 19:739-744.

325. Isobe T, Tsugita A, Okuyama T. The amino acid sequence and the subunit structure of bovine brain S100 protein. J Neurochem 1978; 30:921-923.

326. VanEldik LJ, Zendegin JG, Marshak DR, Watterson DM. Calcium-binding proteins and the molecular basis of calcium action. Int Rev Cytol 1982; 77:1-6.

327. Gaynor R, Irie R, Morton D, Herschmann HR. S-100 protein is present in cultured human malignant melanomas. Nature 1980; 286:400-401.

328. Weiss SW, Langloss JM, Enzinger FM. Value of S-100 protein of soft tissue tumors with particular reference to benign and malignant Schwann cell tumors. Lab Invest 1983; 49:299-308.

329. Hickie RA, Graham MJ, Buckmeier JA, Meyskens FL Jr. Comparison of calmodulin

gene expression in human neonatal melanocytes and metastatic melanoma cell lines. J Invest Dermatol 1992; 99:764-773.

330. Westerman MA, Stoopen GM, van Muijen GN, Kuzincki J, Ruiter DJ, Bloemers HP. Expression of calcyclin in human melanoma cell lines correlates with metastatic behavior in nude mice. Cancer Res 1992; 52:1291-1296.

331. Woodbury RG, Brown JP, Loop SM, Hellström KE, Hellström I. Analysis of normal neoplastic human tissues for the tumor-associated protein p97. Int J Cancer 1981; 27:145-149.

332. Woodbury RG, Brown JP, Yeh M-Y, Hellström I, Hellström KE. Identification of a cell surface protein p97, in human melanomas and certain other melanomas. Proc Natl Acad Sci USA 1981; 77:2183-2187.

333. Brown JP, Woodbury RR, Hart CE, Hellström I, Hellström KE. Quantitative analysis of melanoma-associated antigen p97 in normal and neoplastic tissue. Proc Natl Acad Sci USA 1981; 78:539-543.

334. Brown JP, Nishiyama K, Hellström I, Hellström KE. Structural characterization of human melanoma-associated antigen p97 with monoclonal antibodies. J Immunol 1981; 127:539-546.

335. Brown JP, Hewick RM, Hellström I, Hellström KE, Doolittle RF, Dreyer WJ. Human melanoma-associated antigen p97 is structurally and functionally related to transferrin. Nature 1982; 296:171-173.

336. Rose TM, Plowman GD, Teplow DB, Dreyer WJ, Hellström KE, Brown JP. Primary structure of the human melanoma-associated antigen p97 (melanotransferrin) deduced from the mRNA sequence. Proc Natl Acad Sci USA 1986; 83:1261-1265.

337. Baker EN, Baker HM, Smith CA, Stebbins MR, Kahn M, Hellström KE, Hellström I. Human melanotransferrin (p97) has only one functional iron-binding site. FEBS Lett 1992; 298:215-218.

338. Garratt RC, Jhoti H. A molecular model for the tumor-associated antigen, p97, suggests a Zn-binding function. FEBS Lett 1992; 305:55-61.

339. Smolle J, Soyer HP. Histochemical determinations of copper, zinc, and iron in pigmented nevi and melanoma. Am J Dermatopathol 1991; 13:575-578.

340. Herlyn M, Mancianti ML, Jambrosic K, Bolen JB, Koprowski H. Regulatory factors that determine growth and phenotype of normal human melanocytes. Exp Cell Res 1988; 179:322-331.

341. Herlyn M, Malkowicz SB. Regulatory pathways in tumor growth and invasion. Lab Invest 1991; 65:262-271.

342. Quax PHA, van Muijen GNP, Weening-Verhoeff EJD, Lund LR, Danø K, Ruiter DJ, Verheijen JH. Metastatic behavior of human melanoma cell lines in nude mice correlates with urokinase-type plasminogen activator, its type-1 inhibitor, and urokinase-mediated matrix degradation. J Cell Biol 1991; 115:191-199.

343. Meissauer A, Kramer MD, Schirrmacher V, Brunner G. Generation of cell surface-bound plasmin by cell-associated urokinase-type or secreted tissue-type plasminogen activator: A key event in melanoma cell invasiveness in vitro. Exp Cell Res 1992; 199:179-190.

344. Herlyn D, Iliopoulos D, Jensen PJ, Parmiter A, Baird J, Hotta H, Ross AH, Jambrosic J, Koprowski H, Herlyn M. In vitro properties of human melanoma cells metastatic in nude mice. Cancer Res 1990; 50:2296-2302.

345. Kirchheimer JC, Wojta J, Christ G, Binder BR. Functional inhibition of endogenously produced urokinase decreases cell proliferation in a human melanoma cell line. Proc Natl Acad Sci. USA 1989; 86:5424-5428.

346. Woessner JF Jr. Matrix metalloproteinases and their inhibitors in connective tissue remodeling. FASEB J 1991; 5:2145-2154.

347. Stetler-Stevenson WG. Type IV collagenases in tumor invasion and metastasis. Cancer Metastasis Rev 1990; 9:289-303.

348. Tsushima H, Ueki A, Matsuoka Y, Mihara H, Hopsu-Havu VK. Characterization of a cathepsin-H-like enzyme from a human melanoma cell line. Int J Cancer 1991; 48:726-732.

349. Mueller BM, Reisfeld RA, Edgington TS, Ruf W. Expression of tissue factor by melanoma cells promotes efficient hematogenous metastasis. Proc Natl Acad Sci USA 1992; 89:11832-11836.

350. Bizik J, Lizonová A, Stephens RW, Grófouá M, Vaheri A. Plasminogen activation by t-PA on the surface of human melanoma cells in the presence of α_2-macroglobulin secretion. Cell Reg 1990; 1:895-905.

351. Menrad A, Speicher D, Wacker J, Herlyn M. Biochemical and functional characterization of aminopeptidase N expressed by human melanoma cells. Cancer Res 1993;53:1450-1455.

352. Valyi-Nagy IT, Shih I-M, Greenstein D, Elder DE, Herlyn M. Spontaneous and induced differentiation of cultured human melanoma cells. Int J Cancer 1993; In press.

353. McEwan M, Parsons PG, Moss DJ. Monoclonal antibody against human tyrosinase and reactive with melanocytic and amelanotic melanoma cells. J Invest Dermatol 1988; 90:515-519.

354. Jimbow K, Miyake Y, Homma K, Yasuda K, Izumi Y, Tsutsumi A, Ito S. Characterization of melanogenesis and morphogenesis of melanosomes by physicochemical properties of melanin and melanosomes in malignant melanoma. Cancer Res 1984; 44:1128-1134.

355. Maeda K, Yamada K, Jimbow K. Development of MoAb HMSA-3 and HMSA-4 against human melanoma melanosomes and their reactivities on formalin-fixed melanoma tissue. J Invest Dermatol 1987; 89:588-593.

356. Akutsu Y, Jimbow K. Development and characterization of a mouse monoclonal antibody, MoAb HMSA-1, against a melanosomal fraction of human malignant melanoma. Cancer Res 1986; 46:2904-2911.

357. Jimbow K, Lee SK, King MG, Hara H, Chen H, Dakour J, Marusyk H. Melanin pigments and melanosomal proteins as differentiation markers unique to normal and neoplastic melanocytes. J Invest Dermatol 1993; 100:259S-268S.

358. Takahashi H, Parsons PG, Favier D, McEwan M, Strutton GM, Akutsu Y, Jimbow K. Complementary expression of melanosomal antigens and constant expression of pigment-independent antigen during the evolution of melanocytic tumors. Virchows Arch A Pathol Anat Histopathol 1990; 416:513-519.

359. Vijayasaradhi S, Bouchard B, Houghton AN. The melanoma antigen gp 75 is the human homologue of the mouse b (BROWN) locus gene product. J Exp Med 1990; 171:1375-1380.

360. Halaban R, Moellmann G. Murine and human b-locus pigmentation genes encode a glycoprotein (gp 75) with catalase activity.

361. Thomson TM, Real FX, Murakami S, Cordon-Cardo C, Old LJ, Houghton AN. Differentiation antigens of melanocytes and melanoma: Analysis of melanosome and cell surface markers of human pigmented cells with monoclonal antibodies. J Invest Dermatol 1988; 90:459-466.

362. Murty VV, Bourchard B, Mathew S, Vijayasaradhi S, Houghton AN. Assignment of the human TYRP (brown) locus to chromosome region 9p23 by nonradioactive in situ hybridization. Genomics 1992; 13:227-229.

363. Chintamaneni CD, Ramsay M, Colman MA, Fox MF, Pickard RT, Kwon BS. Mapping the human CAS2 gene, the homologue of the mouse brown (b) locus, to human chromosome 9p22-pter. Biochem Biophys Res Commun 1991; 178:227-235.

364. Vijayasaradhi S, Doskoch PM, Houghton AN. Biosynthesis and intracellular movement of the melanosomal membrane glycoprotein gp 75, the human b (brown) locus product. Exp Cell Res 1991; 196:233-240.

365. Orlow SJ, Boissy RE, Moran DJ, Pifko-Hirst S. Subcellular distribution of tyrosinase and tyrosinase-related protein-1: Implications for melanosomal biogenesis. J Invest Dermatol 1993; 100:55-64.

366. Kwon BS, Chintamaneni C, Kozak CA, Copeland NG, Gilbert DJ, Jenkins N, Barton D, Francke U, Kobayashi Y, Kim KK. A melanocyte-specific gene, Pmel 17, maps near the silver coat color locus on mouse chromosome 10 and is in a syntenic region on human chromosome 12. Proc Natl Acad Sci USA 1991; 88:9228-9232.

367. Demetrick DJ, Herlyn D, Tretiak M, Creasey D, Clevers H, Donoso LA, Vennegoor CJGM, Dixon WT, Jerry LM. ME491 melanoma-associated glycoprotein family: Antigenic identity of ME491, NKI/C-3, neuroglandular antigen (NDA), and CD63 proteins. J Natl Cancer Inst 1992; 84:422-429.

368. Herlyn M, Koprowski H. Melanoma antigens: Immunological and biological characterization and clinical significance. Ann Rev Immunol 1988; 6:283-308.

369. Hotta H, Ross AH, Huebner K, Isobe M,

Proc Natl Acad Sci USA 1990; 87:4809-4813.

Wendeborn S, Chao MV, Ricciardi RP, Tsujimoto Y, Croce CM, Koprowski H. Molecular cloning and characterization of an antigen associated with early stages of melanoma tumor progression. Cancer Res 1988; 48:2955-2962.

370. Atkinson B, Ernst CS, Ghrist BF, Ross AH, Clark WH Jr, Herlyn M, Herlyn D, Maul G, Steplewski Z, Koprowski H. Monoclonal antibody to a highly glycosylated protein reacts in fixed tissue with melanoma and other tumors. Hybridoma 1985; 4:243-255.

371. Donoso LA, Folberg R, Edelberg K, Arbizo V, Atkinson B, Herlyn M. Tissue distribution and biochemical properties of an ocular melanoma-associated antigen. J Histochem Cytochem 1985; 33:1190-1196.

372. Atkinson B, Ernst CS, Ghrist BF, Herlyn M, Blaszczyk M, Ross AH, Herlyn D, Steplewski Z, Koprowski H. Identification of melanoma-associated antigens using fixed tissue screening of antibodies. Cancer Res 1984; 44:2577-2581.

373. Vennegoor C, Calafat J, Hageman P, van Buitenen F, Janssen H, Kolk A, Rumke P. Biochemical characterization and cellular localization of a formalin-resistant melanoma-associated antigen reacting with monoclonal antibody NKI/C-3. Int J Cancer 1985; 35:287-295.

374. Sikora LK, Pinto A, Demetrick DJ, Dixon WT, Urbanski SJ, Temple W, Jerry LM. Characterization of a novel neuroglandular antigen (NGA) expressed on abnormal human melanocytes. Int J Cancer 1987; 39:138-145.

375. Gruters RA, Calafat J, Vennegoor CJ, Jansen H, Ploegh HL. Structural heteogeneity of a human melanoma-associated antigen. Cancer Res 1989; 49:459-465.

376. Ross AH, Dietzschold B, Jackson DM, Earley JJ Jr, Ghrist BD, Atkinson B, Koprowski H. Isolation and amino terminal sequencing of a novel melanoma-associated antigen. Arch Biochem Biophys 1985; 242:540-548.

377. Dixon WT, Demetrick DJ, Ohyama K, Sikora LK, Jerry LM. Biosynthesis, glycosylation, and intracellular processing of the neuroglandular antigen, a human melanoma-associated antigen. Cancer Res 1990; 50:4557-4565.

378. Boucheix C, Benoit P, Frachet P, Billard M, Worthington RE, Gagnon J, Uzan G. Molecular cloning of the CD9 antigen. A new family of cell surface proteins. J Biol Chem 1991; 266:117-122.

379. Classon BJ, Williams AF, Willis AC, Seed B, Stamenkovic I. The primary structure of the human leucocyte antigen CD37, a species homologue of the rat MRC OX-44 antigen. J Exp Med 1989; 169:1497-1502. [Published erratum, J Exp Med 1990; 172:1007].

380. Angelisova P, Vlcek C, Stefanova I, Lipoldova M, Horejsi V. The human leucocyte surface antigen CD53 is a protein structurally similar to the CD37 and MRC OX-44 antigens. Immunogenetics 1990; 32:281-285.

381. Oren R, Takahashi S, Doss C, Levy R, Levy S. TAPA-1, the target of an antiproliferative antibody, defines a new family of transmembrane proteins. Mol Cell Biol 1990; 10:4007-4015.

382. Szala S, Kasai Y, Steplewski Z, Rodeck U, Koprowski H, Linnenbach AJ. Molecular cloning of cDNA for the human tumor-associated antigen CO-029 and identification of related transmembrane antigens. Proc Natl Acad Sci USA 1990; 87:6833-6837.

383. Gaugitsch HW, Hofer E, Huber NE, Schnabl E, Baumruker T. A new superfamily of lymphoid and melanoma cell proteins with extensive homology to *Schistosoma mansoni* antigen Sm23. Eur J Immunol 1991; 21:377-383.

384. Wright MD, Henkel KJ, Mitchell GF. An immunogenic M_r 23,000 integral membrane protein of *Schistosoma mansoni* worms that closely resembles a human tumor-associated antigen. J Immunol 1990; 144:3195-3200.

385. Herlyn D, Powe J, Guerry D IV, Herlyn M, Koprowski H. Inhibition of human tumor growth by IgG2a monoclonal antibodies correlates with antibody density on tumor cells. J Immunol 1985; 134:1300-1304.

386. Giacomini P, Natali PG, Ferrone S. Analysis of the interactions between human high-molecular-weight melanoma-associated antigens and the monoclonal antibodies to three distinct antigenic determinants. J Immunol 1985; 135:696-702.

387. Ziai MR, Imberti L, Nicotra MR, Badaracco G, Segatto O, Natali PG, Ferrone S. Analysis with monoclonal antibodies of the molecular

and cellular heterogeneity of human high-molecular-weight melanoma-associated antigen. Cancer Res 1987; 47:2474-2480.

388. Garrigues HJ, Lark MW, Lara S, Hellström I, Hellström KE, Wight TN. The melanoma proteoglycan: Restricted expression of microspikes, a specific microdomain of the cell surface. J Cell Biol 1986; 103:1699-1710.

389. Rettig WJ, Real FX, Spengler BA, Biebler JL, Old LJ. Human melanoma proteoglycan: Expression in hybrids controlled by intrinsic and extrinsic signals. Science 1986; 231:1281-1284.

390. de Vries JE, Keizer GD, te Velde AA, Voordouw A, Ruiter D, Rumke P, Spits H, Figdor CG. Characterization of melanoma-associated surface antigens involved in the adhesion and motility of human melanoma cells. Int J Cancer 1986; 38:465-473.

391. Lida J, Skubitz AP, Furcht LT, Wayner EA, McCarthy JB. Coordinate role for cell surface chondroitin sulfate proteoglycan and $\alpha_4\beta_1$ integrin in mediating melanoma cell adhesion to fibronectin. J Cell Biol 1992; 118:431-444.

392. Ross AH, Herlyn M, Ernst CS, Guerry D IV, Bennicelli J, Ghrist BF, Atkinson B, Koprowski H. Immunoassay for melanoma-associated proteoglycan in the sera of patients using monoclonal and polyclonal antibodies. Cancer Res 1984; 44:4642-4647.

393. Harper JR, Bumol TF, Reisfeld RA. Characterization of monoclonal antibody 155.8 and partial characterization of its proteoglycan antigen on human melanoma cells. J Immunol 1984; 132:2096-2104.

394. Bumol TF, Reisfeld RA. Unique glycoprotein-proteoglycan complex defined by monoclonal antibody on human melanoma cells. Proc Natl Acad Sci USA 1982; 79:1245-1249.

395. Bumol TF, Walker LE, Reisfeld RA. Biosynthetic studies of proteoglycans in human melanoma cells with a monoclonal antibody to a core glycoprotein of chondroitin sulfate proteoglycan. J Biol Chem 1984; 259:12733-12741.

396. Sturm RA, Bisshop F, Takahashi H, Parsons PG. A melanoma octamer binding protein is responsive to differentiating agents. Cell Growth Diff 1991; 2:519-524.

397. Scheiber E, Harshman K, Kemler I, Malipiero U, Schaffner W, Fontana A. Astrocytes and glioblastoma cells express novel octamer-DNA binding proteins distinct from the ubiquitous Oct-1 and B cell type Oct-2 proteins. Nucl Acids Res 1990; 18:5495-5503.

398. Scholer HR, Hatzopoulos AK, Balling R, Suzuki N, Gruss P. A family of octamer-specific proteins present during mouse embryogenesis: Evidence for germline-specific expression of an Oct factor. EMBO J 1989; 8:2543-2550.

399. Scholer HR. Octamania: The POU factors in murine development. Trends Genet 1991; 7:323-329.

400. van der Bruggen P, Traversari C, Chomez P, Lurquin C, De Plaen E, Eynde VD, Knuth A, Boon T. A gene encoding antigen recognized by cytolytic T lymphocytes on a human melanoma. Science 1991; 254:1643-1647.

===CHAPTER 6===

MARKERS DISTINGUISHING CELLS FROM DIFFERENT STAGES OF MELANOMA PROGRESSION

L arge series of immunohistological studies have been conducted to define those antigens with MAbs that can distinguish between cells of different stages (Table 32).[1-8] Although a direct multicenter comparison with all currently available markers has not been undertaken, it can already be concluded that some markers not only distinguish cells of different stages but also help to predict disease survival. None of the markers, however, can predict therapy response. The most significant diagnostic markers are b_3 of the vitronectin receptor, ICAM-1, and MUC18.

Besides the upregulation of tumor-associated antigens, significant downregulation can be observed. The most significantly downregulated antigen is the dipeptidyl peptidase (CD26), also termed adenosine deaminase-binding protein and characterized by Houghton and colleagues.[7,8] Dipeptidyl peptidase (CD26) expression (Table 31) is completely lost on melanoma cells, whereas all the other antigens are only quantitatively decreased in expression. None is specific for melanoma. Melanoma cells share these antigens with some normal cells in the tumor stroma, suggesting that malignant cells use the same "tools" as normal cells for growth and invasion (Table 33). Structural aberrations leading to possible functional inactivation are not known.

Table 32. Progression markers in melanoma

Upregulated	Downregulated
Adhesion molecules	
$\alpha_v\beta_3$	$\alpha_6\beta_1$
ICAM-1	
MUC18 (gp 113)	
ECM proteins	
Tenascin	Collagen
	Laminin
Growth factor receptors	
EGF receptor	c-*kit*
Transferrin receptor	
Immune recognition molecules	
HLA class II	HLA class I
	Thy-1
Gangliosides	
GD2	GM3
GD3/GM3 ratio > 1.0	
Growth-related	
Ki67	
Enzymes	Dipeptidyl peptidase (CD26 or ADA-binding protein)[a]

[a]Absent on melanomas.

Table 33. Melanoma-associated antigens that are also present on fibroblasts, endothelial cells, or monocytes

Fibroblasts	Endothelial cells	Monocytes[a]
Aminopeptidase N	Vitronectin receptors	CD44
EGF receptor	$\alpha_v\beta_1$	Aminopeptidase N
Tenascin	$\alpha_v\beta_3$	HLA-DR
(HLA-DR)	MUC18	gp30-50 (ME491)
$\alpha_2\beta_1$	ICAM-1	CALLA
	HLA-DR	gp70
	VCAM-1	Transferrin receptor

[a]Expression on activated cells.

REFERENCES

1. Carrel S, Dore J-F, Ruiter DJ, Prade M, Lejeune FJ, Kleeberg UR, Rümke P, Bröcker EB. The EORTC melanoma group exchange program: Evaluation of a multicenter monoclonal antibody study. Int J Cancer 1991; 48:836-847.
2. Holzmann B, Johnson JP, Kandewitz P, Riethmüller G. In situ analysis of antigens on malignant and benign cells of the melanocyte lineage: Differential expression of two surface molecules gp 75 and p 89. J Exp Med 1985; 161:366-377.
3. Lehmann JM, Holzmann B, Breitbart EW, Schmiegelow P, Riethmüller G, Johnson JP. Discrimination between benign and malignant cells of melanocytic lineage by two novel antigens, a glycoprotein with a molecular weight of 113,000 and a protein with a molecular weight of 76,000. Cancer Res 1987; 47:841-845.
4. De Vries JE, Keizer GD, Te Velde AA, Voordouw A, Ruiter D, Rümke PH, Spits H, Figdor CG. Characterization of melanoma-associated surface antigens involved in the adhesion and motility of human melanoma cells. Int J Cancer 1986; 38:465-473.
5. Elder DE, Rodeck U, Thurin J, Cardillo F, Clark WH Jr, Stewart R, Herlyn M. Antigenic profile of tumor progression in human melanocytic nevi and melanomas. Cancer Res 1989; 49:5091-5096.
6. Herlyn M, Koprowski H. Melanoma antigens: Immunological and biological characterization and clinical significance. Ann Rev Immunol 1988; 6:283-308.
7. Houghton AN, Herlyn M and Ferrone S. Melanoma antigens. In: Balch C, Houghton A, Milton G, Sober A, eds. Cutaneous melanoma. Philadelphia: J.B. Lippincott Company, 1992; pp 130-143.
8. Herlyn M, Menrad A, Koprowski H. Structure, function and clinical significance of human tumor antigens. J Natl Cancer Inst 1990; 82:1883-1889.

CHAPTER 7

CONCLUSIONS

The pathobiology of melanoma is being intensely investigated. Led by the detailed description of the histopathological and clinical features of tumor development and progression, researchers have for the last decade attempted to substantiate the morphological description with evidence for qualitative and quantitative changes at the molecular, biochemical, biological, and immunological levels. These studies have led to the delineation of over 100 genes and/or proteins that contribute to melanoma development and progression. However, none of these has, as a single component, been shown to be etiologically involved. After a long and very slow start, molecular genetics and molecular biology of melanoma now yields information at an accelerating rate. Chromosomes 9 and 1 apparently each have a tumor susceptibility gene. Studies in other malignancies have identified genes specifically involved in tumor development; this tremendously stimulates further research. On the other hand, the clinician and patient await prompt answers to help diagnose and treat melanoma, and they will voice their disappointment if these answers are not delivered as quickly as expected. No one can predict when the first melanoma genes will be identified, but important clues should be available within a year. The search for oncogenes and suppressor genes in melanoma has also (slowly) begun. Several interesting "lead genes" have been identified, n-ras, c-kit, and NF-1, which are among the most promising candidate genes in human melanoma development, although additional information on new genes and detailed studies on the implicated genes are needed. Suitable animal models are also obviously needed. The role of transcription factors and other gene regulators is unknown for melanoma. The studies of transcription factors and signal transduction molecules will be intensified as new data provide clues for the roles of specific genes. Although gene expression studies will help our basic understanding of melanoma development, they will not allow quick translation to the clinical setting.

Studies on melanoma-associated antigens have progressed rapidly in the last decade and the data summarized in Chapter 5 are impressive and represent the largest collection for any human malignancy. Beginning as a body of dissociated information on antigens without biological significance, melanoma antigens are now used to diagnose and treat melanoma. These studies have also led to a better understanding of the biology of melanoma. Molecules with best studied functions are bFGF and vitronectin receptor. Both are under intense investigations as targets in the development of rational therapies. Other candidate antigens that may provide future targets for clinical studies are gangliosides and cytokines. Attempts are also being made to use pigment-related antigens as targets for therapy.

Table 34 lists some questions that warrant further investigations. The continuous inability to effectively treat metastatic melanoma is disappointing. Therefore, the mechanisms of drug resistance in melanoma warrant further study. Although the melanoma research community can be proud of their accomplishments, much work remains to be done and the questions listed in Table 34 are far from being answered. This monograph has summarized the data on research in many laboratories on a devastating disease, but it is also clear that only superficial knowledge of melanoma biology has yet been reached. The coming years should provide more basic information on melanoma biology and the development of more effective therapies.

Table 34. Melanoma: Current questions for future answers

1. Is there a melanoma susceptibility gene?

2. How does UV light contribute to melanoma development?

3. Are nevi precursors of melanoma?

4. Which genes contribute to melanoma development and progression?

5. Do lineage-specific transcription factors regulate gene expression in melanoma?

6. Which proteins and carbohydrates expressed by melanoma cells regulate tumor growth, invasion, and metastasis?

7. What is the regulatory role of paracrine factors from the tumor microenvironment, i.e., endothelium and stroma?

8. Can the malignant phenotype be reversed, e.g., can terminal differentiation apoptosin be induced?

9. What role does the host immune response against melanoma play and can it be modulated to suppress melanoma?

10. Why are melanomas so highly drug resistant?

11. How should a rational drug therapy be designed?

12. Besides clinical and pathohistological examinations, are any markers useful for the diagnosis and assessment of risk of recurrence?

ACKNOWLEDGMENTS

Much of the work summarized in this book coming from our laboratory would have been impossible without the intellectual and practical support of my colleagues at The Wistar Institute and at the Pigmented Lesion Study Group of the University of Pennsylvania. Individuals from either institution that I have collaborated with include Wallace Clark, David Elder, DuPont Guerry, Allan Halpern, Dorothee Herlyn, Hilary Koprowski, Alban Linnenbach, Ulrich Rodeck, Lynn Schuchter, and David Speicher. The fellows in my laboratory, who did most of the work, include Peter Borlinghaus, Maria Laura Mancianti, Roland Kath, Jay Jambrosic, Hans Menssen, Bruce Malkowicz, Istvan Valyi-Nagy, Ie-Ming Shih, Istvan Juhasz, Eric Miller, Andreas Menrad, Mark Nesbit, Peter Soballe. The work was only possible through the dedicated efforts of the laboratory technicians, most recently, Tamara Egner, Michelle Myrga, and Rupa Gosh, and the secretarial assistance of Naomi Desta with the Editorial staff at The Wistar Institute.

The funding for this research was obtained from the National Institutes of Health grants CA-25874, CA-10815, CA-47159, and CA-44877.

INDEX